In just 30 days you can be much slimmer, a lot fitter, looking good and feeling marvellous! The secret? *Slimming Magazine*'s unique diet, exercise and beauty plan.

Devised by experts who know themselves what it is like to have conquered a weight problem, the 30-Day Formula is a daily programme which can be adapted to suit any lifestyle. The diet caters for meat-eaters, vegetarians, keen cooks, lazy cooks, saints and sinners. At the beginning of each week you simply weigh yourself and write the amount you need to lose in the box provided: then the experts tell you what meals you may eat for that week. The beauty of the Formula is that it allows you to set your own dieting pace. If you do well you are allowed a 'naughty day' occasionally, and if you cheat you are given a 'saintly day' penance. All the meals are simple to prepare and there is a choice of lunches to be eaten at home or at work.

The exercise programme, illustrated with superb line drawings, is specially designed to ease you into a regular shape-up routine that will help you to become and *stay* really fit. Then, to add the finishing touch, the Formula's beauty and grooming tips — from basic skin and hair care to practical make-up instruction — will ensure that you look your best. And to boost your self-confidence, and help you to overcome those setbacks which sometimes thwart the most determined dieter, there is weekly advice from *Slimming Magazine*'s consultant psychiatrists.

An important feature of the 30-Day Formula is its foolproof tick-off system. As you eat each meal, successfully complete an exercise, or indulge in a special beauty treatment, you simply tick it off — then you can see that you are making progress! If you sincerely want to be slimmer, more supple and to look and feel good, then this is the plan for you.

D0238918

ACKNOWLEDGEMENTS

Editor: Sybil Greatbatch
Beauty and Grooming: Margaret Ford
Home Economist: Glynis McGuinness

All photographs inside the book, unless otherwise credited, are reproduced courtesy of *Slimming Magazine*.

Black and white drawings by Chen Ling.

Slimming Magazine's
30-DAY FORMULA

Edited by Sybil Greatbatch

PANTHER
Granada Publishing

Panther Books
Granada Publishing Ltd
8 Grafton Street, London W1X 3LA

Published by Panther Books 1985

First published in Great Britain by
André Deutsch Limited 1984

Copyright © 1984 by Slimming Magazine,
S. M. Publications Limited

ISBN 0-586-06427-3

Printed and bound in Great Britain by
Ebenezer Baylis & Son Ltd., Worcester, and London

Set in Century Schoolbook

Contents

Introduction

In just 30 days you can be much slimmer, a lot fitter — and feeling marvellous! The secret? Follow our special diet plan, exercise programme and look-good advice.

The 30-Day Formula has been devised by *Slimming Magazine* experts who *know* what it is like to have conquered a weight problem. Diets have been designed to fit into different lifestyles, with a choice of meat or vegetarian meals each day. Chocolate-lovers and cake-eaters are catered for, and some restaurant meals can easily be incorporated into your diet. There is also a pick-yourself-up system if you occasionally fall by the 'weighside'.

Losing weight is a matter of 'balancing the books'. When your body tots up what calories have come in and what it has burned away in various activities, roughly every 3,500 calories surplus to requirement gets turned into one pound more you. To lose a surplus pound, you must get your body about 3,500 calories 'in debt'. An obvious way — and what sensible dieting does — is to cut your calorie income. But, by being extra active, you can boost the number of calories your body pays out. Because a calorie is simply a measure of energy, 'calorie' and 'energy' mean the same thing. So, if you are very active, this cuts the calories made available to your body's bulging bank account.

The Formula's exercise section is very special. You can tackle it even if you've been very lazy for a *long* time. The shape-up movements build up gradually into a muscle-toning programme that you can continue for as long as you wish — ideally for ever!

Each day, too, there is advice on how to assess your beauty and grooming problems and a special treatment to try. None of the treatments involves purchasing expensive creams and lotions. The Formula is firmly based on the realistically helpful, no-nonsense advice which every reader of *Slimming Magazine* expects.

Being overweight can diminish one's confidence and lead to self-doubt, so each week there's advice from our consultant psychiatrist. Success and luck don't just happen: there's a Formula for them as well!

A unique feature of the 30-Day Formula is the tick-off system. As soon as you have eaten a meal, completed an exercise or tried a special beauty treatment, tick it off. You can then *see* that you are making progress.

Do you need to diet?

Check the chart below and you will see the average ideal weight for someone of your height. Depending on the spread of your basic frame, your weight could easily be 5kg/10lb more or less than this figure. Another excellent indicator of whether you have any excess fat on your body is the pinch test. Stand up straight and see if you can pinch between your finger and thumb any flab around your waist, at the top of your arms, or on your thighs. If you can pinch more than an inch, you have some dieting work to do!

What a woman should weigh

minus footwear weights include 2 to 3lb (or about 1kg) for light indoor clothing

Height		Medium Frame		Height		Medium Frame	
4ft-10	*1.47m*	7st-8	*48kg*	5ft-6	*1.68m*	9st-8	*61kg*
4ft-11	*1.50m*	7st-11	*49.5kg*	5ft-7	*1.70m*	9st-9	*61.5kg*
5ft-0	*1.52m*	8st-0	*51kg*	5ft-8	*1.73m*	9st-12	*62.5kg*
5ft-1	*1.55m*	8st-3	*52.5kg*	5ft-9	*1.75m*	10st-2	*64.5kg*
5ft-2	*1.57m*	8st-7	*54kg*	5ft-10	*1.78m*	10st-5	*66kg*
5ft-3	*1.60m*	8st-9	*55kg*	5ft-11	*1.80m*	10st-10	*68kg*
5ft-4	*1.63m*	8st-12	*56.5kg*	6ft-0	*1.83m*	11st-0	*70kg*
5ft-5	*1.65m*	9st-1	*57.5kg*				

You will be keeping a record of your weight loss as you follow the 30-Day Formula, but remember that getting a proper progress report from scales isn't quite as simple as it may sound. Not all scales are equally truthful, so it's a good idea to try to weigh yourself on the same scales each time. If your bathroom scales are standing on carpet, they could be giving you a reading several pounds lighter than the real amount. Brace yourself and from now on always use them placed on a hard floor or put a board underneath them.

Remember that your weight will naturally vary from time to time, even during one day. That meal or glass of water you swallow weighs exactly as much inside you as it did before you had it. You will get a different reading before and after a lavatory trip too. So it is pointless to weigh yourself too often: once a week is enough. Another reason for not hopping on and off the scales every half-day is that the level of water in your body — it accounts for nearly two-thirds of your weight — varies from time to time. For example, you retain rather more water if you have just eaten something salty. And, due to hormonal changes, women tend to retain extra water for a few days before menstruation; it's a purely temporary gain, but can add several pounds. Don't set too much store, then, by your scales' short-term fluctuations; they can be very misleading.

It's the trend of readings over at least 2 or 3 weeks that will tell the true slimming story.

The diet that lets you choose

Most slimmers start dieting determined to shed 2st by last week! That's why, at the outset, the strictest diets are the most psychologically appealing. If we were to inform you, for instance, that 'on this diet you can indulge in quite a lot of food, and you will keep losing a little bit of weight,' you might find the whole idea rather tame and slightly off-putting in your first flush of wild enthusiasm. In dieting there is certainly something to be said for holding your nose, plunging in at the deep end and getting it all over with as quickly as possible.

The beauty of the 30-Day Formula is that it allows you to set your own dieting pace. The three basic meals a day add up to no more than 1,000 calories. On this number of calories the most stubborn surplus-weight problem will disappear; you don't need to go any lower. If at the start of the diet you don't feel the need to eat all three meals, save up for a 'naughty' day later on when your initial resolve has weakened slightly. Strict 1,000-calorie-a-day dieting can be demanding and some days you will find it easier to keep to this limit than others. On difficult days allow yourself an extra snack from those listed and you won't halt your weight loss.

Basically there are 2 ways of keeping your calories to a slimming level. One way is to stick to the same calorie allowance each day. The alternative is the 'swings and roundabouts' approach. On some days you may eat more calories than on others, as long as your weekly total adds up correctly. Taking advantage of days when it is easy to undereat can be the key to weight control for some people.

Is it necessary to eat breakfast? As you will see from the diet menus, we have called the first meal breakfast/supper. You can choose to eat this meal first thing in the morning, after dinner in the evening, or at any other time of day that you wish. For practical purposes, it is the total number of calories you eat each week which will dictate your weight loss, not the time of day that you eat them or even if you eat more some days than others.

What if you are a nibbler by habit? Even if you are keeping to the 3 basic meals a day, you can adapt the menus to your own way of eating. You will find that many of the light meals and most of the main meals have 2 courses. If you are a nibbler, eat 1 course and leave the other for later when you may feel like a snack. There is no need to struggle *not* to eat between meals if that is the pattern of dieting you enjoy. An ostrich-like attitude to snack-eating can lead to 'amnesia' about illegal nibbles. It is always best to allow for your preferences when embarking on a diet.

For someone in ordinary good health, it's no crime to miss a meal. It makes sense for an overweight women to take advantage of times when she's too busy or occupied to eat. Missing a meal when you don't really feel in need of it, is really a splendidly effortless way to control overall calorie intake.

Avoiding temptation
Your kitchen is the prime danger zone: it presents you with more eating temptations than any other place. As you follow the 30-Day Formula, work at eliminating as many visits to the kitchen as you can. Are you in the habit of writing your shopping lists and letters at the kitchen table? Do you have friendly chats in the kitchen over a cup of coffee (and probably a few biscuits!) or set up your sewing machine there to do those boring mending jobs? If so, you are spending literally hours of the day within hand's reach of food and amid tempting aromas. Carry on that way and you probably won't carry on with your diet!

If you have to buy tempting foods such as biscuits and cakes for the rest of the family, stop leaving them lying around on view on kitchen shelves or in transparent jars. They will be a constant temptation to break your diet, so keep them out of sight. See if you can persuade the family to give up any items you find particularly tempting for a few weeks.

Because the 30-Day Formula lets you choose what to eat each day, it has not always been possible to take care of every leftover. If you don't intend to give any remainders to anyone in the family, remember your freezer. Use your freezer manual for guidance on what you can freeze and make little parcels which can easily be taken out to make up dieting meals later. For example, cut corned beef into 50g/2oz portions or freeze chipolata sausages wrapped in twos. If you are cooking any of the keen cook's recipes you may like to make up more than the single portion given and freeze additional meals for future dieting days. Leftover food lying in an almost empty packet or sitting in the fridge can present you with the temptation to eat it in order to be tidy or because you hate to waste food. Steel yourself to become a little less tidy or economical. Throwing away an item of food may present you with 2 minutes' mental anguish. Leave it in your kitchen and you'll be doing battle with it at least 12 hours a day.

9

The value of exercise

There is only one way in which you can remove surplus fat from your body and that is to consume fewer calories in food than you use up in energy expenditure. You will do this mainly by dieting; but increasing your activity level can certainly help to speed up your weight loss on a diet.

How much difference this makes depends on how much exercise you do and which type of exercise you choose. The best calorie-burning exercises are those which involve moving the whole body from one place to another, as in walking or running, rather than those which require you to remain in the same spot just moving your limbs, as in muscle-toning exercises. The faster you move your body from one place to another, the more calories it consumes. Fast walking uses up more calories than slow walking, and jogging or running will burn up almost twice as many calories as most speeds of walking. To reach the ultimate level of calorie expenditure you need to move your whole body quickly, and then to add another factor, such as moving upwards against the pull of gravity. Running upstairs and skipping produce the highest calorie expenditure per minute of all. The 30-Day Formula exercise programme gets those lazy muscles working and is specially designed to make you move faster every day; and, as you progress through the programme, your calorie-burning potential increases.

Even more important than the calorie-burning effects of exercise are the psychological benefits. These benefits have been increasingly recognized as a key factor in curing weight problems over the past decade. It is now almost universally acknowledged in the medical world that exercise can change moods — and that a reasonably vigorous session of exercise is one of the best methods of lifting a depressed mood. As every slimmer knows, it is those bored, listless and depressed moods which are most likely to put you in danger of diet-breaking. The dieter who exercises regularly is less likely to 'cheat' on her diet and is therefore more likely to shed weight at a speedy rate.

A word of warning, though, if you have any health worries. Please check with your doctor before embarking on an exercise plan. You should be particularly careful if you suffer from high blood pressure or have back problems. Gentle exercising usually has health advantages for everyone, but the more strenuous work-outs aren't for people with health problems.

Why bother with beauty?

As you're getting slimmer and fitter, what about the packaging? The Formula reminds you of all sorts of basic beauty rules and gives you lots of new ideas for looking good and feeling great. Not only this, your beauty programme has hidden advantages. To most women with weight problems, the after-dinner hours of the evening are peak hours of extra-eating temptation.

Late-night snacks are often looked upon as being a reward for having got through the trials and tasks of the day, and another major cause of uncontrolled evening eating is boredom. We have all probably experienced those evenings when the TV programmes aren't very good, we somehow can't get into the books we planned to read, we feel a little bit weary and fatigued but not quite ready for bed. Generally we don't know what to do with ourselves. So we end up pacing about and, if we aren't very careful, opening the fridge door and taking out something to eat just to find something to do. The woman who is frequently bored and has time or unused mental energy on her hands is going to have to tackle that problem before she stands any realistic chance of solving her weight problem.

The 30-Day Formula takes care of evening boredom. Not only is there the exercise session, but each day there is a special beauty treatment to try and a continuing beauty programme to follow. The more you pack into your evening, the less likely it is that you will have time to think about food!

An important aspect of both beauty and diet is learning to relax. You will be doing a relaxer exercise every evening before you go to bed, but for troublesome moments during the day (although we wouldn't recommend you try it in the middle of your office or place of work) make use of the following technique:

To relax, you first tense and then consciously relax the muscles in each area of your body. Start at the extremity of the hands or the feet. Clench your fists, making them as tight and tense as possible for some 10 seconds, then let go. Feel your hands and arms going really limp. Now progress to the top of your head and work gradually downwards. The secret of doing it well is to tense then relax each little bit of you — your eyelids, for instance, by first of all closing them extra tight, your nose by wrinkling it up, your tongue by clamping your jaws and then pushing hard against the roof of your mouth. When you are relaxed you need to fill your mind with something to banish the thought of food. You do this by conjuring up a mental picture of yourself in some particularly pleasant situation. Just any old image won't do: it has to be vivid and detailed enough for you to mentally experience all kinds of pleasurable sensations. Imagine yourself, for example, lying in a cornfield with the summer sun warming your body and a soft breeze rippling through the corn. Got the idea? It's a matter of getting totally involved in an imagined experience. For some people, this mental and physical relaxation banishes all troublesome food cravings. One word of warning, though, if you try this technique. Take care that the image you conjure up isn't one which, in real life, would lead to eating. Otherwise, after taking all this trouble, you might mentally progress to opening your picnic basket and . . . damn, here's that wretched food on your mind again.

How the 30-Day Formula works
Weigh yourself on Day 1 and enter your weight in the space provided. Check your ideal weight and work out how much you need to lose. You will then be directed to either keep to the 3 basic meals a day or to add 1 or 2 snacks. Stick to the planned menus and 2 snacks a day and there's no mistaking the fact that you will be eating no more than 1,500 calories. Almost all women will lose weight if they stick to this calorie allowance, although if you only have a few pounds to lose or if you have been dieting for a long period of time, your weight loss on 1,500 calories may be rather slow. For this reason if you have under 1st to lose, you should keep to the 3-meal menus which will bring your calorie intake down to 1,000 a day.

The menus have been designed to give you a good nutritional balance of foods over each week. You will get the best results if you stick to each day's menu as planned. But if you are an erratic eater, there is no reason why you shouldn't miss a meal and save it for a day when you want to eat more. The tick-off system will ensure that over a week your total calories will average out correctly. If there are any items in a day's menu that you dislike, check the Calorie Swap-Shop on page 265. It may be possible to swap this item for something you'd enjoy more. The swaps are all worked out to give you the same number of calories, but do check weights carefully. If you swap 115g/4oz broad beans for sweetcorn, you'll only get 50g/2oz.

It may be easier to be strict with yourself at the beginning of your diet than later on. If, when you reach the 3rd or 4th week, you start feeling desperate for an extra snack occasionally, be kind to yourself and take advantage of the

fact that your exercise programme will now be making an
extra calorie-burning contribution to your dieting day.

Remember to weigh and measure all foods carefully. For
this you will need a kitchen scale that can cope with small
units, a set of measuring spoons and a jug for liquids. The
only exceptions to this rule are green vegetables, lettuce,
cucumber and cress. If we have not given an exact weight
in a recipe this means you can eat as much as you like of
these very low-calorie vegetables.

You have a daily milk allowance which can be used in tea
or coffee throughout the day or consumed all at once.
Where milk is used in a recipe this is in addition to your
daily allowance. Apart from that you can drink as much
black coffee and tea as you wish, provided that only no-
calorie artificial sweeteners are used. You can also drink low-
calorie squashes and mixers without any restriction. If you
wish to have an alcoholic drink occasionally, you can have
this instead of a snack. Each snack is worth 250 calories and
you will find a list of drinks in the Calorie Chart of Basic
Foods at the back of this book. Because alcoholic drinks don't
contain any nutrients you need and can destroy vitamins
taken from other foods, we don't advise you to drink every
day of the week.

Each day you can save up for a special occasion or plain
'naughty' day. If you do happen to have an uncontrolled
binge one day then you must follow it with a 'Saintly Day'
menu (page 253) the next day to make amends.

At the beginning of each day we give a shopping list so
that you can easily plan to have all the food for your chosen
menu readily available. Shop once a week if you can, which
will save you risking supermarket temptation. If at the end
of your 30 days you still have more weight to lose, you can
repeat the daily menus for as long as you wish.

It is very important to follow your exercise programme
every day so that you gradually build up the sessions. What
you are aiming for is to get into a regular daily exercise
habit that you will enjoy continuing.

If you are overweight the chances are that you'll be
slightly, if not entirely, exercise resistant. This may be
partly psychological: stemming from embarrassing
occasions in the school gym, from a lack of confidence in
your own ability that has grown with your weight worries,
or just plain laziness. The programme has been specially
devised to build up your exercise confidence and to show
you that you don't have to join an exercise class or squash
club to increase your activity level. As you progress
through the exercise programme, you can break the

exercises down into shorter sessions as long as you complete them all by the end of the day.

Your beauty and grooming plan should also be followed on a daily basis. If, however, you are too busy doing other things to fit in, say, a facial, then you can do it another evening. But do resist the temptation not to do a treatment just because you don't feel like it. That sort of excuse can lead to the biscuit barrel. Your beauty and grooming plan has been designed to make your skin feel softer, to improve your make-up techniques and to identify and care for your beauty problem areas, so that at the end of the 30- day programme you should feel more confident in every way and know that you are looking your best.

Week 1

☐☐ Weigh yourself and write in your weight here

☐☐ Now check the chart on page 7 and write in your ideal weight here

☐☐ Write in the amount you have to lose here

Now tick one of these boxes, and this is your menu plan for this week

☐ If you have under 1st to lose, you can have breakfast/supper, a light meal and a main meal each day.

☐ If you have between 1st and 3st to lose, you can have breakfast/supper, a light meal, a main meal and one snack.

☐ If you have over 3st to lose, you can have breakfast/supper, a light meal, a main meal and two snacks.

Shopping Checklist Day 1

First choose your meals, then write by each relevant item the amount you require. You will not need all the items listed.

Amount required	Amount required	Amount required
Fruit and Vegetables	**Dairy Produce/Eggs**	Oil-free French
Cabbage	Cheddar cheese	dressing
Carrots	Edam or Tendale	Salt and pepper
Cauliflower	cheese	Sultanas or raisins
Celery	Eggs	Tomato ketchup
Cucumber	Low-fat spread	Yeast extract
Garlic (optional)	Natural yogurt	
Grapes	Skimmed milk	
Mushrooms	(or dried low-fat	
Onions	milk powder)	
Tomatoes	**Grocery**	
Watercress	Bran breakfast	
Apples	cereal	
Bananas	Crispbreads	
Cooking apples	Wholemeal bread	
Pears	**Store cupboard**	
Frozen Foods	Artificial sweetener	
Broccoli or	Beef stock cube	
runner beans	Cornflour	
Peas	Lemon juice	
Meat, Poultry and Fish	Low-calorie salad	
Chipolata sausage	dressing	
Chicken	Mixed herbs	
Lamb loin chop	Mustard	
Streaky bacon	Nutmeg or cinnamon	

Diet Day 1

☐ *275ml/½ pint skimmed milk or reconstituted low-fat powdered milk*

Measure milk into a jug and use for tea and coffee throughout the day. You can drink as much tea and coffee as you wish, with milk from your allowance or black. You may use artificial sweeteners, but do not sweeten drinks with sugar.

BREAKFAST/SUPPER MEAL

Either ☐ *2 tomatoes, grilled without fat; 1 rasher streaky bacon, well grilled; 1 small slice wholemeal bread, 25g/1oz*

Or ☐ *2 eggs, size 3, scrambled with 15ml/1 tablespoon skimmed milk (extra to allowance); 1 tomato, grilled without fat*

Or ☐ *25g/1oz any bran breakfast cereal, eg: Honey Bran, All Bran, Bran Buds, Bran Flakes, Sultana Bran, Bran Muesli or Farmhouse Bran; 75ml/5 tablespoons skimmed milk (extra to allowance); 6 grapes*

LIGHT MEAL

Either to eat at home
Chicken with Vegetables plus Fruit

☐ *225g/8oz chicken leg joint* *115g/4oz carrots, fresh or*
25g/1oz onion *frozen*
Mixed herbs *115g/4oz peas, frozen*
1 small apple

Discard skin from chicken and place joint on a piece of foil. Chop onion and place on chicken, then sprinkle with mixed herbs. Make into a parcel and bake at 200°C/400°F, gas mark 6, for 30 minutes. Boil vegetables and serve with chicken. Follow with apple.

Or to take to work
Chicken Salad plus Fruit

☐ *75g/3oz roast chicken meat* *30ml/2 tablespoons low-*
Watercress *calorie salad dressing*
Cucumber *1 medium apple*
Celery *1 medium pear*

Discard any skin from chicken and slice meat into thin strips. Make a salad with as much watercress, sliced cucumber and celery as you wish, and mix with chicken. Add salad dressing just before eating. Follow with fruit.

Or if you prefer to eat vegetarian Crunchy Carrot Salad plus Banana

2 medium carrots
75g/3oz red or white cabbage
1 stick celery
2 spring onions
15ml/1 level tablespoon sultanas or raisins
30ml/2 tablespoons oil-free French dressing
15ml/1 tablespoon lemon juice
Salt and pepper
2 crispbreads
10ml/2 level teaspoons low-fat spread
1 medium banana

Grate the carrots; finely shred cabbage; finely chop celery and slice onions thinly. Mix all vegetables in a bowl and stir in the raisins. Add the dressing and lemon juice and mix well. Season to taste. Serve with crispbreads and low-fat spread. Follow with banana. The salad can be taken to work in a plastic container. Wrap the crispbreads separately.

MAIN MEAL

Either a quick recipe Mixed Grill plus Stewed Apple

150g/5oz lamb loin chop
1 beef or pork chipolata sausage
2 rashers streaky bacon
115g/4oz mushrooms
1 tomato
115g/4oz broccoli or runner beans, frozen
175g/6oz cooking apple
Artificial sweetener to taste
Pinch nutmeg or cinnamon

Remove any fat from chop and well grill with sausage and bacon. Poach mushrooms in a little stock or water. Halve tomato and grill. Boil broccoli or beans and serve with mixed grill. Peel and slice apple and stew with a little water and nutmeg or cinnamon. Add artificial sweetener after cooking.

Or a keen cook's recipe Saucy Lamb Chop plus Baked Apple

150g/5oz lamb loin chop
½ onion
5ml/1 level teaspoon low-fat spread
½ clove garlic (optional)
½ beef stock cube
175ml/6floz water
10ml/2 level teaspoons tomato ketchup
Pinch mixed dried herbs
10ml/2 level teaspoons cornflour
115g/4oz carrots
115g/4oz peas, frozen
175g/6oz cooking apple
15ml/1 level tablespoon sultanas or raisins
Artificial sweetener (optional)

Cut any visible fat from chop. Finely chop onion. Melt low-fat spread in a non-stick pan, add onion and cook for a minute, stirring. Crush the garlic and add to saucepan with stock cube, water, tomato ketchup and herbs. Bring to the boil, cover and simmer for 15 minutes. Blend cornflour with a little cold water, stir into the sauce. Bring to the boil, cook for 2 minutes, stirring constantly. Add a little extra water if necessary to prevent sauce sticking. Well grill chop. Boil vegetables and serve with lamb chop and herby sauce. Core the apple and cut the skin around the middle. Stand the apple in an ovenproof dish and fill the cavity with dried fruit. Place 30ml/2 tablespoons water in the dish and bake at 180°C/350°F, gas mark 4, for 30 minutes. Serve with artificial sweetener if required.

Or if you prefer to eat vegetarian
Herby Cauliflower Cheese and Mushrooms

225g/8oz cauliflower
15g/½oz low-fat spread
15g/½oz cornflour
150ml/¼ pint skimmed milk
50g/2oz Cheddar cheese with herbs or plain, grated
Salt and pepper
1.25ml/¼ level teaspoon prepared mustard
30ml/1 rounded tablespoon fresh breadcrumbs
50g/2oz button mushrooms

Break the cauliflower into florets and cook in boiling salted water until just tender — about 10 minutes. Drain and place in an ovenproof dish and keep warm. Place the low-fat spread, cornflour and skimmed milk in a saucepan and bring to the boil, stirring continuously. Cook for 2 minutes. Reserve 30ml/1 rounded tablespoon grated cheese and add the remainder to the sauce. Season with salt and pepper and the mustard and stir well. Pour over the cauliflower. Mix the reserved cheese with the breadcrumbs and sprinkle on top. Brown under a moderate grill. Poach the mushrooms in a little lightly salted water or stock. Drain and serve with the cauliflower.

Snack 1

1 small carton low-fat natural yogurt
1 large banana
1 medium apple

Either eat individually or cut up fruit and mix with yogurt.

Snack 2

3 crispbreads
15ml/1 level tablespoon yeast extract
40g/1½oz Edam or Tendale cheese
1 tomato

Spread crispbreads with yeast extract and top with sliced or grated cheese and tomato slices.

If you completed the day without cheating at all, tick here and move on to Day 2.

If you cheated, do a 'Saintly Day' tomorrow (page 253) instead of the set menu.

☐ If you do not eat one meal or snack that you are allowed, tick this box and save up for a 'Naughty Day'. When you have two ticks saved, you can do any of the Thoroughly Naughty Day's Menus *instead* of your next day's diet.

Exercise Day 1

MORNING *When you wake up, sit on the edge of the bed with your hands by your sides.*

Exercise 1 ☐ Lift arms, keeping them straight with palms facing upwards, bend elbows and link fingers behind head. Stretch up with fingers linked and palms upward, so that you can feel your spine elongating. Breathe in through your nose as you stretch up and out through your mouth as you lower your arms to original position.

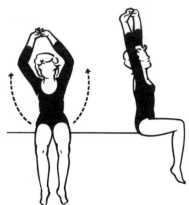

Repeat 5 times

Even if you haven't yet opened your eyes, you can continue with the next exercise.

Exercise 2 ☐ Sit up straight and drop head forward so that your chin rests on your chest. Circle the head slowly round to the right, extend to the back and circle round to the left, finishing in the original position with your head on your chest.
Repeat 4 times circling to the right

☐ Repeat 5 times circling to the left

That nasty neck-crunching noise is all yesterday's tension coming out

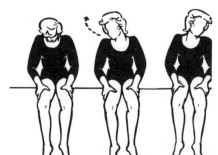

Exercise 3 ☐ Cross legs and slightly raise up the right foot. Circle foot, just moving the ankle, 5 times to the left and 5 times to the right.

☐ Repeat with left foot.

That is the end of your first exercise session — it wasn't too painful, was it? You may not exactly bounce into the bathroom but you'll certainly be in a positive state of mind to start your day.

LUNCHTIME ☐ Walk for 5 minutes in any direction. Turn and return the same way, but this time do the same distance in 4 minutes.

Yes, that really is all you have to do. Easy, wasn't it?

EVENING ☐ Stand at the bottom of a flight of stairs (about 15 steps) and run to the top. Walk down again.
This is a very strenuous exercise and you should not do it if you are very overweight or if you have high blood pressure. Alternatively, you may:

☐ Run on the spot for 1 minute lifting feet well off the floor.

Bedtime Relaxer ☐ Lie flat on your back on the bed or on the floor, with your arms down by your sides. Inhale as you lift up your arms and bring them over your head until they rest on the floor or bed behind you. Clench your hands into fists and push your buttocks up as you tense and stretch every muscle in your body, including facial muscles. Hold for a count of 5 then breathe out and relax body. Keep arms over your head and relax fingers, legs, feet, head and let all tensions drain away.

Beauty Shopping List Week 1

The number of items you will require depends on your skin type and problems. Check through the week's treatments and write down the products you need to purchase.

All-purpose cream,	Cuticle cream	Nail polish remover
baby cream or	Eggs	Nail scissors
rich skin cream	Emery board	Oatmeal
Almond oil	Face pack	Orange
Bath oil	Honey	Salt
Body lotion	Lemon juice	Skin cream
Cleanser	Manicure stick	10-volume peroxide
Cotton wool	Moisturizer	Toner

Beauty Day 1

Today's special treatment
You start your beauty programme with an all-over skin softening treatment.

If you have sensitive skin ☐ Relax in a warm bath to which you have added a few drops of almond oil, bath oil, or a few drops of milky skin cleanser. Squeeze out a flannel and rub gently over body.

If you have an oily skin ☐ This 'spring clean' for your skin will whisk away dry particles, leaving your skin silky, slightly tingly and fresh. The massage cream below contains salt, so be careful that you don't use it on sensitive areas or on any cuts. Although it won't harm you, it could be very uncomfortable.

Massage Cream Recipe *1 teaspoon salt*
1 tablespoon skin cream or almond oil

This recipe is enough for covering an average-size body. If you are larger than average, increase the quantity.

Mix salt with cream or oil and spread lightly onto skin, using circular movements with the fingers. You'll probably find that it is best to stand in the bath while you are doing this. Work upwards from ankles to thighs and over body, then massage from the wrists to shoulders. But stop there. This treatment is not for the neck or face, and any tiny broken veins should be strictly avoided. When you are well oiled and covered in cream, shower off or take a dip in warm water, working up a good lather. Rinse well and splash with cold water, or as cold as you can bear it.

If you have dry skin

Do a body massage exactly as for oily skin, using the same recipe. Then dry yourself and cover your body or dry areas with body lotion or cream.

Shopping Checklist Day 2

Choose your meals, then write in by each relevant item the amount you require.

Amount required	Amount required	Amount required
Fruit and Vegetables	**Dairy Produce/Eggs**	Marmalade
Carrots	Cheddar cheese	Mixed herbs
Chicory	Eggs	Oil-free French
Cucumber	Low-fat spread	dressing
Green pepper	Natural low-fat	Salt and pepper
Mushrooms	yogurt	Stock cube
Onion	Skimmed milk	Tomato purée
Potatoes	**Grocery**	
Tomatoes	Baked beans	
Watercress	Bran breakfast	
Banana	cereal	
Grapefruit	Cashew nuts	
Grapes	or peanuts	
Lemon	Currant bun	
Orange	Pasta shells	
Pineapple	Pineapple canned in	
Frozen Foods	natural juice	
Beefburgers	Potato crisps	
Mixed peas and	Rice	
carrots	Wholemeal bread	
Mixed peas and	**Store cupboard**	
sweetcorn	Dried thyme	
Meat, Poultry and Fish	or marjoram	
Prawns	Cornflour	
Stewing beef	Low-calorie salad	
	dressing	

Diet Day 2

☐ 275ml/½ pint skimmed milk or reconstituted low-fat powdered milk.

BREAKFAST/SUPPER MEAL

Either ☐ 1 egg, size 3, boiled; 1 small slice wholemeal bread, 25g/1oz; 5ml/1 level teaspoon low-fat spread

Or ☐ 25g/1oz any bran breakfast cereal; 75ml/5 tablespoons skimmed milk (extra to allowance); 6 grapes

Or ☐ 2 small slices wholemeal bread, 25g/1oz each, toasted; 10ml/2 level teaspoons low-fat spread; 10ml/2 level teaspoons marmalade

LIGHT MEAL

Either to eat at home **Poached Egg on Toast with Beans**
☐ 1 egg, size 3   150g/5.3oz can baked beans
1 small slice wholemeal bread, 25g/1oz
Poach egg in water or in a non-stick poacher without fat. Serve on toasted bread with heated baked beans.

Or to take to work **Prawn and Pasta Salad**
☐ 115g/4oz peeled prawns, fresh or frozen   Watercress
Chicory
25g/1oz pasta shells, raw   30ml/2 tablespoons oil-free
Cucumber   French dressing
Allow frozen prawns to defrost. Boil pasta until cooked and rinse under cold water. Chop as much cucumber, watercress and chicory as you wish and mix with drained pasta and prawns. Pour on French dressing just before eating.

Or if you prefer to eat vegetarian **Pasta and Fruit Salad**
☐ 1 small grapefruit   15ml/1 tablespoon low-calorie
1 small orange   salad dressing
1 ring pineapple, fresh or canned in natural juice   30ml/2 tablespoons natural low-fat yogurt
25g/1oz pasta shells, raw
Peel and segment grapefruit and orange and cut into small pieces. Cut pineapple into chunks. Boil pasta until cooked, then drain, rinse and drain again. Mix pasta with fruit. Stir salad dressing into yogurt, then mix with pasta salad.

Either a quick recipe **Beefburgers and Vegetables plus Fruit and Yogurt**

2 beefburgers, 50g/2oz each
115g/4oz mixed peas and carrots, frozen
115g/4oz mushrooms
½ stock cube
115g/4oz grapes
15ml/1 tablespoon low-fat yogurt, any flavour

Well grill beefburgers. Boil peas and carrots and poach mushrooms in water with stock cube. Serve vegetables with beefburgers. Follow with grapes and yogurt.

Or a keen cook's recipe **Beef Stew and Vegetables plus Orange**

75g/3oz very lean stewing beef
1 medium carrot
1 small onion
25g/1oz mushrooms
10ml/2 level teaspoons cornflour
½ stock cube
150ml/¼ pint boiling water
15ml/1 level tablespoon tomato purée
Salt and pepper
Pinch mixed herbs
115g/4oz potato
115g/4oz mixed peas and sweetcorn, frozen
1 large orange

Cube the beef, discarding any visible fat. Dice the carrot and onion; put into a saucepan with beef and mushrooms. Mix the stock cube with boiling water and pour half over the meat and vegetables. Mix cornflour with a little cold water and stir in remaining stock. Pour into saucepan, stirring. Add the tomato purée, seasoning and herbs, then cover and bring to the boil. Simmer for about 1 hour until the meat is tender. Boil the vegetables and serve with beef stew. Follow with orange.

Or if you prefer to eat vegetarian **Vegetable and Nut Risotto**

½ small onion
1 small green pepper
2 tomatoes
50g/2oz brown long-grain rice
225ml/8fl oz boiling water
1.25ml/¼ level teaspoon dried thyme or marjoram
25g/1oz mushrooms
Salt and pepper
Little grated lemon rind
25g/1oz salted cashew nuts or peanuts

Chop the onion; remove seeds from pepper and chop flesh; peel and chop tomatoes. Put into a shallow pan with rice. Add the boiling water and herbs. Bring to the boil, stir well then cover and simmer gently for 35 minutes. Add chopped mushrooms and extra water, if necessary. Season to taste with salt and pepper and stir in the grated lemon rind. Cover and continue to simmer for 5 minutes or until the rice is tender and the water is absorbed. Just before serving stir in nuts.

Snack 1

1 small packet crisps, any flavour
25g/1oz Cheddar cheese

Snack 2 ☐ *1 currant bun, 50g/2oz*   *1 small banana*
*10ml/2 level teaspoons low-
    fat spread*

☐ If you completed the day without cheating at all, tick here
and move on to Day 3.

☐ If you cheated, do a 'Saintly Day' tomorrow (page 253)
instead of the set menu.

☐ If you do not eat one meal or snack that you are allowed,
tick this box and save up for a 'Naughty Day'. When
you have two ticks saved,you can do any of the Thoroughly
Naughty Day's Menus *instead* of your next day's diet.

Exercise Day 2

MORNING ☐ Repeat Excrcise 1: 5 times

☐ Repeat Exercise 2: 5 times to right
5 times to left

☐ Repeat Exercise 3: 5 times circling left and right with
right foot
5 times circling left and right with left foot.

Exercise 4 ☐ Stand upright with feet slightly
apart. Stretch hands above head
then try to touch the floor between
your feet. Repeat 5 times.
*Bend knees slightly. It doesn't
matter if you can't reach the floor
to begin with. You will gradually
find that it gets easier.*

LUNCHTIME ☐ Walk for 6 minutes. Turn and return the same way in 5
minutes.
*Try to pick a route that doesn't mean crossing a lot of main
roads. Standing on the curb waiting for traffic to pass
doesn't count as walking.*

EVENING ☐ Run to the top of the stairs and down again.

Or ☐ Jog on the spot for 2 minutes.

Remember to do your running up and down stairs either in bare feet or non-slip shoes. And do a double check that there is no loose carpet or anything to trip over.

Bedtime Relaxer ☐

Beauty Day 2

Well, we all have something to hide. Some problems can be prevented, and most can be camouflaged. Before you try today's special treatment, check the following list. Tick the problems which apply to you, then read how you can tackle them. Do you have:

☐ Broken veins (*spider naevi*)?

☐ Goosepimples?

☐ Rough, wrinkled or discoloured elbows?

☐ Dingy areas inside thighs or under arms?

Spider naevi
These are tiny dark 'broken' veins which show up mauvely through the skin, often as a result of being overweight. Professional treatment may disperse them but there's no guarantee. Favourite locations are face and thighs, areas to be treated with utmost care. No hot baths, cold rinses, strong astringent lotions. No highly-seasoned dishes and the minimum of social drinking. Use a cover-up make up to protect and disguise them. More details of this are given on page 188, Day 22.

Goosepimples
This is the name given to roughened skin which stays permanently 'pimply' and is usually found on tops of arms and over bottom and thighs. It's a sign of sluggish circulation, so stimulate by massaging with soap and a soft brush (a shaving brush or toothbrush), working up a lather.

Splash with cold water, pat dry and rub in cream or body lotion. Do this every other day for the first week, and once or twice a week after that until skin is smooth. Do not use this treatment though, on areas where there are broken veins.

Elbows

Elbows easily become rough, wrinkled or discoloured and that's hardly surprising. Think of the work that skin has to do here, stretching and contracting to accommodate arm movements. Lighten elbows the lazy way, by resting them in lemon halves which have been squeezed and used for cooking. Try it next time you settle down for a good read. Or mix lemon juice with a little salt and rub in. Rinse off after 5 to 10 minutes and palm in cream. Aim for twice-weekly treatment.

Defeat dinginess

The skin on the inside of thighs or under arms often becomes discoloured and to counteract this, blend hand cream with 6 drops of 10-volume peroxide and smooth it in once or twice a week, but not for 24 hours before or after shaving, or after using a depilatory cream for hair removal. More about that on page 87, Day 10.

Today's special treatment

A long, languid massage before bed, but after taking a bath or shower when the skin is soft and receptive. Use a little body lotion and stroke it upwards from tops of feet, along calves and up over thighs. Then upwards from wrists to shoulders. Finally, from tops of thighs to neck, except over breasts. Feel your body glow, and feel the skin growing silkier. Enjoy the sensation. It's the next best thing to a professional massage — especially if you can get your nearest and dearest to do it for you.

And before we go on . . . a few ground rules

Get plenty of sleep. Skin and hair show the strain of late nights and tired eyes lack lustre.

Don't panic if things go a little wrong. When things seem 'too much', stop dashing. Just long enough to take a few deep breaths.

Forget 'why me?' Because every woman has her problems. If you *feel* defeated, you will *look* defeated, and move and react in a downbeat way. You acted positively by deciding to read this book. Don't spoil the mood. Stick with it!

Know Your Skin Tomorrow you will start facial treatments and you will need to know how dry or oily your skin is. Tomorrow morning do a simple test with a large tissue. Press it firmly over your face first thing in the morning before you wash. Then examine it for oiliness.

Oily ☐ If there are extensive oily patches you can assume you have an oily skin, so tick this box.

Combination ☐ An oily central strip only, suggests that you have combined oily and dry patches.

Normal ☐ A trace of oil at the centre shows that your skin is normal.

Dry ☐ If the tissue is oil-free, your skin is dry.

Shopping Checklist Day 3

Choose your meals, then write in by each relevant item the amount you require.

Amount required	*Amount required*
Fruit and Vegetables	Eggs
Carrots	Fruit yogurt
Celery	Low-fat spread
Mustard and cress	Skimmed milk
Onion	**Grocery**
Potato	Bran breakfast
Tomatoes	cereal
Apple	Butter beans
Banana	Crispbreads
Grapefruit	Lentils
Grapes	Wholemeal bread
Orange	**Store cupboard**
Peach	Chutney
Frozen Foods	Mustard
Broad beans	Salt and pepper
Individual mousse	Tomato sauce
Peas and sweetcorn	Yeast extract
Runner beans	
Meat, Poultry and Fish	
Chipolata sausage	
Boiled ham	
Chicken joint	
Dairy Produce/Eggs	
Cottage cheese	
Edam or Tendale cheese	

Diet Day 3

☐ 275ml/½ pint skimmed milk or reconstituted low-fat powdered milk

BREAKFAST/SUPPER MEAL

Either ☐ 25g/1oz any bran breakfast cereal; 75ml/5 tablespoons skimmed milk (extra to allowance); 6 grapes

Or ☐ 2 tomatoes, grilled without fat; 1 beef or pork chipolata sausage, well grilled; 1 small slice wholemeal bread, 25g/1oz

Or ☐ 1 slice wholemeal bread, 40g/1½oz; 1 egg, size 3; 5ml/1 level teaspoon low-fat spread
Dip bread in beaten egg and fry in a non-stick pan greased with low-fat spread.

LIGHT MEAL

Either to eat at home
Cottage Cheese on Toast plus Banana

☐ 1 small slice wholemeal bread, 25g/1oz   Mustard and cress
50g/2oz cottage cheese   1 medium banana
½ peach, fresh or well-drained canned
Toast bread and top with cottage cheese and chopped peach. Serve with as much mustard and cress as you wish. Follow with banana.

Or to take to work
Cheese and Cress Sandwich plus Fruit

☐ 2 small slices wholemeal bread, 25g/1oz each   Mustard and cress
50g/2oz cottage cheese   1 small apple
Make sandwich with cottage cheese and mustard and cress. Take apple to eat afterwards.

MAIN MEAL

Either a quick recipe
Chicken and Vegetables plus Mousse

☐ 225g/8oz chicken joint   15ml/1 level tablespoon
115g/4oz potato   chutney or tomato sauce
115g/4oz peas and   Individual frozen mousse,
sweetcorn, frozen   about 50g/2oz, any variety
Grill chicken joint and remove skin. Boil vegetables and

serve with chicken and chutney or tomato sauce. Follow with mousse.

Or a keen cook's recipe
Ham Pudding and Vegetables

115g/4oz lean boiled ham
2 tomatoes
40g/1½oz wholemeal bread
5ml/1 level teaspoon made mustard
75ml/3floz skimmed milk
1 egg, size 3
Salt and pepper
115g/4oz runner beans
115g/4oz broad beans

Discard any visible fat from ham and cut lean meat into triangles. Put into a small ovenproof dish and cover with tomato slices. Spread mustard onto bread and cut into triangles. Place bread on top of tomato. Mix together milk, egg and seasonings and pour into dish. Bake at 180°C/350°F, gas mark 4, for 20 minutes until the pudding is just set. Serve with boiled beans.

Or if you prefer to eat vegetarian
Lentil Stew and Green Beans plus Mousse

50g/2oz lentils
275ml/½ pint vegetable stock or water
1 small onion
1 medium carrot
2 sticks celery
2.5ml/½ level teaspoon yeast extract
50g/2oz canned butter beans
Salt and pepper
115g/4oz runner beans
1 individual frozen mousse, any brand or flavour

Wash lentils and put in a pan with the stock or water. Bring to the boil, reduce heat, cover and simmer gently for 30 minutes. Add the sliced onion and carrot, and chopped celery. Stir in yeast extract. Cover and simmer for a further 30 minutes. Stir in butter beans; season to taste with salt and pepper and heat through. Serve with boiled green beans. Follow with mousse.

Snack 1

1 medium grapefruit
1 small orange
1 fruit yogurt, any flavour

Either eat separately or make the following cocktail. Cut grapefruit in half, remove flesh and cut into cubes. Peel and segment orange and add to grapefruit. Mix with yogurt and spoon back into grapefruit halves.

Snack 2

3 crispbreads
15ml/1 level tablespoon yeast extract
40g/1½oz Edam or Tendale cheese
1 tomato

Spread yeast extract on crispbreads. Top with cheese and tomato.

☐ If you completed the day without cheating at all, tick here and move on to Day 4.

☐ If you cheated, do a 'Saintly Day' tomorrow (page 253) instead of the set menu.

☐ If you do not eat one meal or snack that you are allowed, tick this box and save up for a 'Naughty Day'. When you have two ticks saved, you can do any of the Thoroughly Naughty Day's Menus *instead* of your next day's diet.

Exercise Day 3

MORNING ☐ Repeat Exercise 1: 5 times

☐ Repeat Exercise 2: 5 times to right
5 times to left

☐ Repeat Exercise 3: 5 times circling left and right with right foot
5 times circling left and right with left foot
Make sure you're not waggling that leg. Make nice big circles from the ankle only.

☐ Repeat Exercise 4: touch the floor 10 times

LUNCHTIME ☐ Walk for 7 minutes. Turn and return the same way in 6 minutes.

EVENING ☐ Run to the top of the stairs and down again, then up again and walk down.
Take a rest if you wish when you reach either the top or the bottom of the stairs. You don't burn up more calories by staying out of breath.

Or ☐ Jog on the spot for 3 minutes.

Bedtime Relaxer ☐

Beauty Day 3

Face Basics

Skin is naturally good at taking care of itself. Oil secreted by sebaceous glands keeps it soft and supple, sweat glands contribute moisture and millions of tiny cells from the skin's outer layer are constantly being renewed. So why do we need to bother with skin care? Two reasons. One is that the natural process does not always work as effectively as it should; and secondly, skin has to be defended against unfair everyday wear and tear. When skin produces too much natural oil — sebum — the tiny openings become blocked. The sebum hardens and produces a blackhead which may erupt into a spot. You can read how to cope with this and other blemishes on page 42, Day 4. When there is too little natural oil, the skin is left dry and taut and it becomes drier with cold winds, central heating and too much sun. It may also be irritated by grime in the surrounding air. So you can see why normal skin needs routine protection. It needs cleansing, it may need moisturizing; but what it doesn't normally need is an elaborate daily ritual with a lot of costly creams.

Cleansing

Cleansing is important morning and night, and especially at night. If you prefer to use soap and water, choose a mild soap, such as one of the baby varieties. A cosmetic cleanser dissolves make-up more effectively and may suit a dry skin better.

Buying guide: creams and thicker fluids for drier skin; gels or clear liquids for oily skin, or a milky cleanser which can be used on part dry, or part oily skin.

Toning

Toning lotions are slightly bracing. They whisk off cleanser and leave the face feeling fresh. There are astringent, spiritous lotions to cope with oily skin, but lotions for dry skins are milder and often labelled 'fresheners'.

For a home-made toner use 2 parts of rosewater to 1 of witch hazel for dry skin. Or 2 parts of witch hazel to 1 part rosewater for oily skin. A chemist will mix this for a small charge.

Moisturizing

Moisturizers are light creams or lotions which soften skin

and help it retain moisture in the way that natural oil does. Moisturize after cleansing and toning.

How to cleanse and care
Smooth cleanser over skin with fingers or cotton wool or lather lightly with soap and water upwards from neck. Work in well over chin, nose and around nostrils. Fingerprint gently around eyes. Wipe off cleanser with cotton wool or rinse off lather. Apply toner with fingers or cotton wool. Then moisturize. Follow the arrows in the sketch.

Today's special treatment

For dry and mbination skins: your own home salon massage

First cleanse your skin. Then squeeze out a clean face flannel in hand-hot water and press it over your face. Massage with baby oil or a few drops of the oil mixed with moisturizer. Use finger tips to stroke it firmly over neck and face, following the arrows in the sketch. Go gently round eyes, finger-printing lightly with third finger. Reheat flannel, lay over your face until it begins to cool. Relax for 10 minutes. Wipe off residue of oil and cream. Splash face with cool water or toner.

Skin very oily and spotty?
Omit this treatment and do the steam and lather treatment tomorrow. Instead you can work on some of those problem areas:

Elbows
Mix lemon juice with a little salt and rub into discoloured elbows. Rinse off after 5 to 10 minutes and apply body lotion.

Goosepimples?
Lather goosepimply areas with a soft brush. Splash with cold water, pat dry and rub in cream or body lotion.

Dinginess?
Blend hand cream with 6 drops of 10-volume peroxide and smooth it into dingy areas on thighs and under arms.

Shopping Checklist Day 4

Choose your meals, then write in by each relevant item the amount you require.

Amount required	*Amount required*
Fruit and Vegetables	Corn snacks
Courgettes	Low-calorie
Onion	tomato soup
Potatoes	Muesli or fruit
Tomatoes	and nut bar
Banana	Onion sauce mix
Grapes	Rice
Orange	Wholemeal bread
Peach	**Store cupboard**
Pear	Flour
Frozen Foods	Mixed herbs
Courgettes	Salt and pepper
Meat, Poultry and Fish	Stock cube
Calves' or lamb's	Vegetable oil
liver	
Streaky bacon	
Dairy Products/Eggs	
Cottage cheese	
Edam or Tendale	
cheese	
Eggs	
Low-fat spread	
Skimmed milk	
Grocery	
Bran breakfast	
cereal	

Diet Day 4

☐ 275ml/½ pint skimmed milk or reconstituted low-fat powdered milk

BREAKFAST/SUPPER MEAL

Either ☐ 2 tomatoes, grilled without fat, 1 rasher streaky bacon, well grilled; 1 small slice wholemeal bread, 25g/1oz

Or ☐ 1 egg, size 3, boiled; 1 small slice wholemeal bread, 25g/1oz; 5ml/1 level teaspoon low-fat spread

Or ☐ 25g/1oz any bran breakfast cereal; 75ml/5 tablespoons skimmed milk (extra to allowance); 6 grapes

LIGHT MEAL

Either to eat at home
Soup, Cheese on Toast and Fruit

☐ 1 can low-calorie tomato soup, any brand — 25g/1oz Edam or Tendale cheese
1 small slice wholemeal bread, 25g/1oz — 1 tomato — 1 small orange or peach

Heat soup. Toast bread on one side. Top with sliced tomato and grated cheese. Grill until cheese bubbles. Follow with fruit

---

Or to take to work
Soup, Cheese Sandwich and Fruit

☐ 1 can low-calorie tomato soup, or 1 packet instant low-calorie tomato soup, any brand — 2 small slices wholemeal bread, 25g/1oz each
50g/2oz cottage cheese
1 tomato
1 small orange or peach

Take tomato soup to work in a vacuum flask or make up instant soup with boiling water. Make a sandwich with bread, cottage cheese and sliced tomato. Take fruit to eat afterwards.

MAIN MEAL

Either a quick recipe
Grilled Liver, Rice and Vegetables plus Fruit

☐ 115g/4oz calves' or lamb's liver — 115g/4oz courgettes, fresh or frozen
2 rashers streaky bacon — 2 tomatoes
30ml/2 level tablespoons raw rice — 1 medium pear

Grill liver and well grill bacon. Boil rice and courgettes. Grill halved tomatoes and serve with liver, bacon, rice and vegetables. Follow with pear.

Or a keen cook's recipe
Liver Provençal plus Fruit

☐

115g/4oz calves' or lamb's liver	*Pinch mixed herbs*
10ml/2 level teaspoons flour	*1 tomato*
Salt and pepper	*30ml/2 level tablespoons raw rice*
1 small onion	
5ml/1 teaspoon oil	*115g/4oz courgettes, fresh or frozen*
150ml/¼ pint stock, made with ½ stock cube	*1 medium pear*

Cut the liver into strips and put into a small polythene bag with flour, salt and pepper. Shake well to coat liver. Chop onion. Heat oil in a non-stick pan and add onion and liver (shake off any excess flour). Brown the liver on both sides then reduce heat. Stir in stock and herbs, simmer gently for 10 minutes. Skin and chop tomato and add to liver. Heat through. Boil the rice and courgettes and serve with liver. Follow with a pear.

Or if you prefer to eat vegetarian
Potato, Cheese and Onion Bake plus Pear

☐

115g/4oz new potatoes, raw or canned	*Half a 275ml/½ pint packet onion sauce mix*
115g/4oz tomatoes	*150ml/¼ pint skimmed milk*
Salt and pepper	*1 medium pear*
25g/1oz Edam or Tendale cheese	

Cook the raw potatoes in salted water until just tender and drain. Slice potatoes and put half at the bottom of a small ovenproof dish. Cover with half the tomato slices and season. Cover with the grated cheese. Top with remaining tomato and potato slices. Make up the onion sauce with the skimmed milk as instructed and pour over vegetables. Bake at 220°C/425°F, gas mark 7 for 30 minutes. Follow with a pear.

Snack 1

☐

1 small packet corn snacks, any flavour	*25g/1oz Edam cheese*

Snack 2

☐

1 individual muesli or fruit and nut bar	*1 medium banana*

☐ If you completed the day without cheating at all, tick here and move on to Day 5.

☐ If you cheated, do a 'Saintly Day' tomorrow (page 253) instead of the set menu.

☐ If you do not eat one meal or snack that you are allowed, tick this box and save up for a 'Naughty Day'. When you have two ticks saved, you can do any of the Thoroughly Naughty Day's Menus *instead* of your next day's diet.

Exercise Day 4

MORNING ☐ Repeat Exercise 1: 5 times

☐ Repeat Exercise 2: 5 times to right
5 times to left

☐ Repeat Exercise 3: 5 times circling left and right with right foot
5 times circling left and right with left foot

☐ Repeat Exercise 4: touch the floor 15 times
Stretch up really tall before you bend. If you can't yet touch the floor with your fingers, just get down as far as you can.

LUNCHTIME ☐ Walk for 8 minutes. Turn and return the same way in 7 minutes.

EVENING ☐ Run to the top of the stairs and down again twice.

Or ☐ Jog for 4 minutes.
Remember to keep lifting your knees up when you're jogging. If it gets boring running on the spot, jog around the house or into the garden.

Bedtime Relaxer ☐

Beauty Day 4

If you are plagued with spots it's no comfort to be told they're probably 'hormonal' and will eventually disappear. You won't want to wait that long. Fight back.

Blackheads
Blackheads are the most common troublemakers — tiny plugs of sebum which have hardened and darkened and can become septic and erupt into a spot. What to do: fill a bowl with very hot water. Drape a towel over your head to form a 'tent' and steam face for about 5 minutes until the water begins to cool. Work up a lather with a complexion brush or *soft* toothbrush using a mild soap. Rinse off, splash with cold water. Dab antiseptic on blackhead areas. Do this twice a week for a fortnight. Obstinate blackheads may need to be pressed out after steaming, but remember to wrap your fingers in tissues.

Relaxed pores
These are often called 'open' pores. They respond to the soap and water brushing described above, but there is no need to steam. You can buy cleansing grains or 'pore grains'; these provide gentle friction and are a useful way of budging tiny blackheads which sometimes prove difficult to remove. Follow the manufacturer's directions carefully.

Spots
Spots may persist in dry skin. They will sometimes appear around the chin pre-menstrually. Dab with antiseptic. If an angry spot has a white head it can be pierced with a sterilized needle which has been passed through a flame and dipped in antiseptic. Then press the spot gently with a tissue and apply antiseptic or calamine lotion.

Acne
You will know if you have it. Spots, blackheads, oily skin and misery. There are medicated, oil-reducing treatments which help and a chemist can advise. There are also treatments available on a doctor's advice which help you to cope while camouflaging. For other spot cover-ups, see page 187, Day 22.

Today's special treatment
Facial pack for smoothing skin ☐ Buy a face pack to suit your skin type or try one of these

home-brewed beauty treats. Leave a space around the eyes when applying the face pack. Moisturize after removing pack unless your skin is oily.

Oat cooler for dry, sensitive skin Two teaspoons of fine oatmeal mixed to a paste with a little boiling water. When cool, spread over face. Rinse off after 10 minutes.

Honey softener for dry or normal skin Add a few drops of squeezed orange juice to a tablespoon of honey. Warm slightly and spread over face. Remove with moistened cotton wool after 15-20 minutes. Rinse off with warm water; splash with cool.

Egg flip for oily skin Add a little fresh lemon juice to the white of an egg and beat to a stiff froth. Paint on to face with a pastry brush. Rinse off with warm water after 15-20 minutes. Cool rinse.

Shopping Checklist Day 5

Choose your meals, then write in by each relevant item the amount you require.

Amount required		Amount required		Amount required	
Fruit and Vegetables		Low-fat natural		Tomato purée	
Apple		yogurt		Worcestershire sauce	
Banana		Low-fat spread		Yeast extract	
Carrot		Skimmed milk			
Celery		**Grocery**			
Leek		Bran breakfast			
Melon		cereal			
Onion		Canned tomatoes			
Orange		Crispbreads			
Potato		Currant bun			
Tomato		Dried apricot halves			
Frozen Foods		Instant dried potato			
Broad beans		Spaghetti in			
Peas		tomato sauce			
Runner beans		White sauce mix			
Sweetcorn		Wholemeal bread			
Meat, Poultry and Fish		Wholemeal roll			
Cod fillet		**Store cupboard**			
Liver pâté or		Ground mace			
garlic sausage		Low-calorie			
Dairy Products/Eggs		seafood sauce			
Cheese spread		Marmalade			
Edam or Tendale		or jam			
cheese		Mustard			
Eggs		Salt and pepper			
		Stock cube			

Diet Day 5

☐ *275ml/½ pint skimmed milk or reconstituted low-fat powdered milk*

BREAKFAST/SUPPER MEAL

Either ☐ *2 eggs, size 3, scrambled with 15ml/1 tablespoon skimmed milk (extra to allowance); 1 tomato, grilled without fat*

Or ☐ *25g/1oz any bran breakfast cereal; 75ml/5 tablespoons skimmed milk (extra to allowance); 2 dried apricot halves, chopped*

Or ☐ *2 small slices wholemeal bread, 25g/1oz each, toasted; 10ml/2 level teaspoons low fat spread; 10ml/2 level teaspoons marmalade or jam*

LIGHT MEAL

Either to eat at home
Pâté and Toast plus Fruit

☐

50g/2oz liver pâté or garlic sausage
1 small slice wholemeal bread, 25g/1oz, toasted

1 tomato, sliced
1 medium apple or orange

Or to take to work
Pâté and Crisp-bread plus Fruit

☐

50g/2oz liver pâté or garlic sausage
2 crispbreads

2 tomatoes
1 medium apple or orange

Or if you prefer to eat vegetarian
Vegetable Soup and Roll

☐

1 medium carrot
1 small onion
1 stick celery
1 leek
115g/4oz canned tomatoes
5ml/1 level teaspoon tomato purée

400ml/¾ pint vegetable stock
Salt and pepper
Pinch of ground mace
5ml/1 teaspoon yeast extract
1 wholemeal roll

Wash or peel vegetables, then coarsely grate the carrot, finely chop the onion and celery and finely slice the leek. Chop the canned tomatoes. Place all vegetables in a pan with tomato purée, stock, salt and pepper to taste, mace and yeast extract. Bring to the boil, cover and simmer for about 25 minutes. Check seasoning and add more if necessary. Serve hot with roll. The soup can be taken to work in a vacuum flask.

Either a
quick recipe
Grilled Cod
and Vegetables

175g/6oz cod fillet
5ml/1 level teaspoon low-fat
 spread
150g/5oz potato
15ml/1 tablespoon skimmed
 milk

115g/4oz runner beans
115g/4oz sweetcorn
15ml/1 level tablespoon
 low-calorie seafood sauce

Grill the cod fillet topped with low-fat spread. Boil potato
and mash with skimmed milk. Boil beans and sweetcorn and
serve with cod, seafood sauce and mashed potatoes.

Or a keen
cook's recipe
Fish Pie
and Vegetable
plus Melon

115g/4oz cod fillet
150ml/¼ pint skimmed milk
50g/2oz peas, frozen
150ml/¼ pint boiling water
½ packet white sauce mix

60ml/4 level tablespoons
 instant dried potato
1 tomato
200g/7oz melon

Poach the cod in milk. When fish is cooked, drain off milk
and reserve. Flake the fish and put into an individual
ovenproof dish. Boil peas. Make up white sauce as
instructed on packet using reserved milk. Add peas to sauce
and pour over fish. Make up potato with boiling water and
put into a piping bag. Pipe potato around the edge of the
dish (or spoon it round). Heat pie under grill until the
potato is slightly browned. Decorate with quartered tomato.
Melon can be eaten as a starter or dessert.

Or if you
prefer to eat
vegetarian
Spaghetti and
Tomato Au
Gratin

213g/7½oz can spaghetti in
 tomato sauce
1 tomato
25g/1oz Edam or Tendale
 cheese

60ml/4 tablespoons fresh
 wholemeal breadcrumbs
115g/4oz broad beans
1 medium apple

Heat the spaghetti in tomato sauce, then transfer to a small
ovenproof dish. Cover with sliced tomato. Mix grated
cheese and breadcrumbs together. Sprinkle over tomato.
Heat under a hot grill until cheese melts and browns. Boil or
heat broad beans and serve with spaghetti. Follow with apple.

Snack 1

1 currant bun, 50g/1¾oz
10ml/2 level teaspoons low-
 fat spread

1 small banana

Snack 2

20ml/4 teaspoons
 Worcestershire sauce
60ml/4 tablespoons low-fat
 natural yogurt
10ml/2 teaspoons tomato
 purée

2.5ml/½ teaspoon prepared
 mustard
Raw vegetables of your
 choice
2 crispbreads
2 triangles cheese spread

Mix together Worcestershire sauce, yogurt, tomato purée and mustard. Use it as a dip for vegetables. Spread crispbreads with cheese spread.

☐ If you completed the day without cheating at all, tick here and move on to Day 6.

☐ If you cheated, do a 'Saintly Day' tomorrow (page 253) instead of the set menu.

☐ If you do not eat one meal or snack that you are allowed, tick this box and save up for a 'Naughty Day.' When you have two ticks saved, you can do any of the Thoroughly Naughty Day's Menus *instead* of your next day's diet.

Exercise Day 5

MORNING ☐ Repeat Exercise 1: 5 times

☐ Repeat Exercise 2: 5 times to right
5 times to left

☐ Repeat Exercise 3: 5 times circling left and right with right foot
5 times circling left and right with left foot

☐ Repeat Exercise 4: touch the floor 15 times

Exercise 5 ☐ Stand with feet slightly apart. Lift up right arm, keeping it straight, to above head. Bend over to left sliding left hand down leg, bending as far as you can go. Move from waist only, keeping feet on floor. Straighten up and drop arms to side.

47

Repeat with left arm bending to right. Repeat these 2 movements 4 more times.

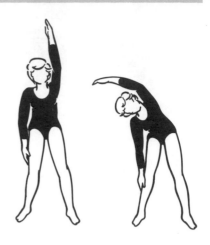

LUNCHTIME Walk for 9 minutes. Turn and return the same way in 8 minutes.
Make sure the first part of your walk is nice and brisk so that you have to push yourself a bit to get back to your starting place in the faster time.

EVENING Run to the top of the stairs and down again twice. Then jog on the spot for 1 minute.

Or Jog on the spot or around the house and garden for 6 minutes.

Bedtime Relaxer

Beauty Day 5

Keep fresh

Let's face it, could there be anything more embarrassing than to be singled out as someone who is decidedly 'not nice to be near'?

Personal freshness is something we take for granted. But just as some people have a greater weight problem, others have a heavier output of perspiration. Everyone perspires: up to 4 pints every 24 hours, pumped from around 2 million sweat glands. Some sweat is secreted by larger apocrine glands and contains fatty acids and body waste. These glands are situated where sweat cannot easily evaporate: under arms, vaginal area, soles of feet. Their output is often accelerated by tension or excitement.

Protection
Most people need protection other than regular bathing.
Deodorants help check odour but not wetness. They are
mild, and useful for a sensitive skin. Anti-perspirants help
in blocking under-arm perspiration. They won't impede the
body's automatic cooling system because perspiration over
the rest of the body is not affected. Anyone who perspires
freely — younger and more active people, anyone with an
oily skin — will need an anti-perspirant.

The right anti-perspirant for you?
Most are roll-ons or sprays. A roll-on may give better
coverage but products vary in strength. If you are unable to
find one which works for you, why not ask the advice of
your local chemist's shop? They will be able to tell you the
best-selling brands and others which are formulated to
solve the problems of excessive perspiration.

'It doesn't work as well as it used to'
That's because the body can build up a resistance. This can
be overcome by switching brands or alternating between
two different types of anti-perspirant. There are soaps
which contain a deodorizing ingredient and have a slight
delaying action on odour-producing bacteria. Talcs absorb
moisture; they won't prevent perspiration but they make
skin feel more comfortable and soothe any soreness.
Perspiration increases with added pounds but normally
stabilizes when this is dieted away.

Today's special treatment
For a silky neck you will need a rich skin cream or an all-
purpose or baby cream. Wring out a small hand towel in
hand-hot water and wrap it around your neck. Remove the
towel before it cools and stroke cream firmly but gently
upwards over neck, from collar bone to chinline.
　　Rewarm the towel, wrap again, and rewarm towel as it
cools. If you have a microwave oven put it in there to rewarm for a few seconds. After 15-20 minutes splash neck
with cool water. Some extra advice for neck care can be
found on page 105, Day 13.

Goosepimples?　Lather goosepimply areas with a soft brush. Splash with
cold water, pat dry and rub in cream or body lotion.

Cleanse, tone　Cleanse, tone and moisturize your face in the morning and
moisturize　at night.

Shopping Checklist Day 6

Choose your meals, then write in by each relevant item the amount you require.

Amount required	Amount required	Amount required
Fruit and Vegetables	Edam or Tendale	Vinegar
Carrot	cheese	Yeast extract
Celery	Eggs	
Courgette	Low-fat	
Cucumber	fruit yogurt	
Mustard and cress	Low-fat	
Onion	natural yogurt	
Potato	Low-fat spread	
Tomatoes	Skimmed milk	
Apple	**Grocery**	
Banana	Apricots in	
Pear	natural juice	
Tangerine or	Baked beans in	
mandarin orange	tomato sauce	
Frozen Foods	Bran breakfast cereal	
Individual mousse	Crispbreads	
Peas	Rice	
Meat, Poultry and Fish	Wholemeal bread	
Chipolata sausage	**Store cupboard**	
Lamb or pork chop	Cornflour	
Pork fillet	Horseradish sauce	
Roast beef	Low-calorie	
Dairy Produce/Eggs	salad dressing	
Cottage cheese	Piccalilli	
with chives	Salt and pepper	
	Stock cube	

Diet Day 6

☐ 275ml/½ pint skimmed milk or reconstituted low-fat powdered milk

BREAKFAST/SUPPER MEAL

Either ☐ 2 tomatoes, grilled without fat; 2 beef or pork chipolata sausages, well grilled; 1 small slice wholemeal bread, 25g/1oz

Or ☐ 25g/1oz any bran breakfast cereal; 75ml/5 tablespoons skimmed milk (extra to allowance); 1 tangerine or mandarin orange

Or ☐ 1 slice wholemeal bread, 40g/1½oz; 1 egg, size 3; 5ml/1 level teaspoon low fat spread
Dip the bread in beaten egg and fry in a non-stick pan greased with low-fat spread.

LIGHT MEAL

Either to eat at home
Beef Open Sandwich plus Pear
☐ 1 slice rye or wholemeal bread, 40g/1½oz
5ml/1 level teaspoon horseradish sauce
50g/2oz lean roast beef
Cucumber
1 tomato
1 pear
Spread bread with horseradish sauce. Top with beef and sliced cucumber and tomato. Follow with pear.

Or to take to work
Roast Beef Sandwich
☐ 2 small slices wholemeal bread, 25g/1oz each
10ml/2 level teaspoons horseradish sauce
50g/2oz lean roast beef
Cucumber
1 tomato
Spread bread with horseradish sauce and make a sandwich with beef and cucumber. Take tomato to work separately and eat with sandwich.

Or if you prefer to eat vegetarian
Egg and Cress Roll
☐ 1 wholemeal bread roll
1 egg, size 3
15ml/1 tablespoon low-calorie salad dressing
Mustard and cress
Hard boil egg, then chop and mix with salad dressing. Spread on roll and fill with as much mustard and cress as you wish.

Either a quick recipe
Chop with Beans plus Mousse

175g/6oz lamb or pork chop
150g/5.3oz can baked beans in tomato sauce

1 individual frozen mousse, any brand or flavour

Remove all visible fat from chop and well grill. Heat beans and serve with chop. Follow with mousse.

Or a keen cook's recipe
Pork Fillet with Apricots and Vegetable

75g/3oz pork fillet
½ small onion
Salt and pepper
115ml/4floz stock, made with stock cube
5ml/1 level teaspoon cornflour

227g/8oz can apricots in natural juice
5ml/1 teaspoon vinegar
30ml/2 tablespoons rice, raw
115g/4oz peas, frozen
30ml/2 tablespoons low-fat natural yogurt

Discarding any visible fat, cube the pork and chop the onion. Put into a saucepan and season. Add stock and bring to boil. Mix cornflour with 2 tablespoons apricot juice and add to meat, stirring. Add vinegar. Cover and simmer for about 40 minutes until pork is tender. Add a little more stock or water if necessary to prevent sticking. Add 3 apricot halves and heat through. Boil rice and peas and mix together. Serve with pork and apricots. To follow, serve remaining apricots topped with natural yogurt.

Or if you prefer to eat vegetarian
Cheesy Baked Potato and Vegetable Medley

200g/7oz potato
Salt and pepper
50g/2oz cottage cheese with chives
30ml/2 level tablespoons Piccalilli
15g/½oz Edam or Tendale cheese

1 small onion
1 small carrot
1 courgette
1 stick celery
2 tomatoes
1 individual low-fat fruit yogurt

Scrub potato and bake at 200°C/400°F, gas mark 6, for about 1 hour until soft. Cut in half lengthwise and scoop out centre. Mash potato with cottage cheese and season to taste. Pile back into potato cases. Top each half with a tablespoon of Piccalilli and sprinkle grated Edam or Tendale on top. Return to oven until the cheese has melted. Chop onion, dice the carrot, slice courgette. Boil until just cooked. Drain and add chopped celery and tomato and heat through. Serve with baked potato. Follow with yogurt.

Snack 1

1 small carton natural low-fat yogurt

1 large banana
1 medium apple

Eat individually or cut up fruit and mix with yogurt.

Snack 2 ☐
2 crispbreads
10ml/2 teaspoons yeast
extract

40g/1½oz Edam or Tendale
cheese
2 tomatoes

Spread crispbreads with yeast extract. Top with cheese and tomatoes.

☐ If you completed the day without cheating at all, tick here and move on to Day 7.

☐ If you cheated, do a 'Saintly Day' tomorrow (page 253) instead of the set menu.

☐ If you do not eat one meal or snack that you are allowed, tick this box and save up for a 'Naughty Day'. When you have two ticks saved, you can do any of the Thoroughly Naughty Day's Menus *instead* of your next day's diet.

Exercise Day 6

MORNING ☐ Repeat Exercise 1: 5 times

☐ Repeat Exercise 2: 5 times to right
5 times to left

☐ Repeat Exercise 3: 5 times circling left and right with right foot
5 times circling left and right with left foot

☐ Repeat Exercise 4: touch the floor 15 times

☐ Repeat Exercise 5: bend to the left and right 10 times
When you bend sideways, allow yourself to bounce a little then try to push that arm further down the leg. Really feel the stretch right down your side.

LUNCHTIME ☐ Walk for 10 minutes. Turn and return the same way in 8 minutes.
As your walks get longer, you need to take extra care to wear suitably comfortable shoes. If you go to work, keep a spare pair of walking shoes there.

EVENING ☐ Run to the top of the stairs and down again twice. Jog on the spot for 2 minutes.

Or ☐ Jog for 7 minutes.

Bedtime Relaxer ☐

Beauty Day 6

Hands deserve a round of applause. They are mobile, strong and yet so sensitive, capable of performing the most intricate movements. Much of this is due to their structure: around 30 bones within each hand and wrist, augmented by tiny 'sesame seed' bones within the tendons of the thumb. Their repertoire is amazing; they can deliver a karate chop or touch a rose petal without bruising it. Hands are good at keeping up appearances, considering the punishment they get. How many times do you dip yours in water, dowse them in detergent, expose them to the wear and tear of housework or pound the keys of a typewriter? But when the skin roughens and nails break, they soon respond to a little extra care.

Hand care
This basically is commonsense. Rinse off detergent, avoid very hot water and, ideally, use hand cream each time you dry your hands. Smooth in hand cream as if drawing on tight gloves, stroking hands from fingertip to wrist and between fingers. Work it into tips and base of nails to give them a bonus. And, yes, it is a bore to have to pull on protective plastic gloves for wet chores; but if your hands are rough and dry and your nails are fragile, it may be the only way to fight back. Sprinkle talc inside plastic gloves and they should slide off more easily. Remove the gloves as soon as work's done, as they can make your hands sweat and irritate the skin.

Today's special treatment
☐ For your manicure you will need: cotton wool; nail polish remover; an emery file; cuticle cream for split cuticles; a towel or tissue to dry nails; manicure stick and nail scissors to cope with hangnails; small bowl or basin containing warm soapy water. For extra kindness add 2 teaspoons of hair

conditioner to the water. Are your nails very fragile or flaky? Then use warm baby oil instead of soapy water for soaking. Warm it by placing the bottle in hot water with the cap loosened. Pour 4 tablespoons into a finger bowl or small basin.

☐ 1. Rub nail polish remover on all nails using cotton wool. Remove polish, one nail at a time, working in a circular direction. Take care to remove polish from around cuticles.

☐ 2. File nails one way only, as see-saw movements encourage splitting. File from sides to centre, rounding off nail tip. Avoid filing nails low down at sides or they will split. Use the darker side of the emery file to start with, then finish with a whisk over with the finer, lighter side.

☐ 3. Massage cuticle cream into cuticles.

☐ 4. Soak nails for 5 minutes in the water or oil. Dry nails or wipe away traces of oil.

☐ 5. Wrap a wisp of cotton wool around the end of the manicure stick and *very* gently scrape around cuticles to remove any flakes of skin or other debris. Carefully trim off loose skin or hangnails. Draw the manicure stick behind nail tips without applying pressure.

☐ 6. Dip fingers in water; flutter them and dry. Check that all loosened skin has disappeared from around cuticles.

☐ 7. Massage in hand cream.

☐ 8. If you are applying nail polish, turn to page 132, Day 16.

Elbows ☐ Still rough or discoloured? Mix lemon juice with a little salt and rub in. Rinse off after 5 to 10 minutes and apply body lotion.

Dinginess? ☐ Blend hand cream with 6 drops of 10-volume peroxide and smooth it into dingy areas on thighs or under arms.

Cleanse, tone moisturize ☐ Cleanse, tone and moisturize your face in the morning and at night.

Shopping Checklist Day 7

Choose your meals, then write in by each relevant item the amount you require.

Amount required	*Amount required*	*Amount required*
Fruit and Vegetables	**Dairy Produce/Eggs**	Mint sauce
Carrots	Butter	Oil-free French
Cauliflower	Cheese spread	dressing
Celery	Eggs	Salt and pepper
Courgettes	Low-fat natural yogurt	Stock cube
Cucumber	Low-fat powdered milk	Sweet pickle
Mushrooms	Low-fat spread	Tomato purée
Onion	Skimmed milk	Vegetable oil
Potato	**Grocery**	Yeast extract
Tomatoes	Bran breakfast cereal	
Apple	Brown long-grain rice	
Apricot	Crispbreads	
Banana	Peaches or apricots,	
Cooking apple	canned in low-calorie	
Orange	syrup or juice	
Peach	Peanut butter	
Frozen Foods	Raisins	
Ice cream	Red kidney beans	
Mixed vegetables	Sweetcorn	
Runner beans	Wholemeal bread	
Sweetcorn	**Store cupboard**	
Meat, Poultry and Fish	Cornflour	
Chipolata sausage	Curry powder	
Leg of lamb	Dried thyme	
Roast lamb	Honey	
Streaky bacon	Lemon juice	

Diet Day 7

☐ *275ml/½ pint skimmed milk or reconstituted low-fat powdered milk*

BREAKFAST/SUPPER MEAL

Either ☐ *2 tomatoes, grilled without fat; 2 rushers streaky bacon, well grilled; 1 small slice wholemeal bread, 25g/1oz*

Or ☐ *1 egg, size 3, boiled; 1 small slice wholemeal bread, 25g/1oz; 5ml/1 level teaspoon low-fat spread*

Or ☐ *25g/1oz any bran breakfast cereal; 75ml/5 tablespoons skimmed milk; 15ml/1 level tablespoon raisins*

LIGHT MEAL

Either to eat at home
Sausage and Mash

☐ *2 beef or pork chipolata sausages*   *Salt and pepper*
150g/5oz potato   *115g/4oz runner beans*
15ml/1 tablespoon skimmed milk   *15ml/1 level tablespoon sweet pickle*

Well grill the sausages. Boil potatoes and mash with skimmed milk and seasoning to taste. Boil beans and serve with sausage, mash and pickle.

Or to take to work
Sausage and Bean Salad plus Yogurt

☐ *1 beef or pork chipolata sausage*   *25g/1oz red kidney beans, canned*
1 stick celery   *15ml/1 tablespoon oil-free French dressing*
Cucumber
25g/1 oz sweetcorn, frozen or canned   *1 small carton low-fat natural yogurt*

Well grill the sausage and slice. Slice celery and dice cucumber. Mix with sweetcorn, kidney beans and sausage. Toss in oil-free French dressing. Follow with a natural yogurt.

Or if you prefer to eat vegetarian
Creamy Mushrooms and Cheese on Toast

☐ *115g/4oz button mushrooms*   *10ml/2 level teaspoons cornflour*
10ml/2 level teaspoons low-fat powdered milk   *2 small slices wholemeal bread, 25g/1oz each*
115ml/4floz water or vegetable stock   *2 triangles cheese spread, 15g/½oz each*
Salt and pepper

Wash the mushrooms and place in a saucepan. Dissolve the skimmed milk powder in the water or stock and pour over mushrooms. Bring to the boil, cover and simmer for 5 minutes. Blend the cornflour with a little cold water and add to mushrooms. Boil for 1 minute or until thickened and season to taste. Toast the bread on both sides. Spread with cheese and pile the creamy mushrooms on top.

MAIN MEAL

Either a quick meal **Roast Lamb and Vegetables**

115g/4oz roast lamb, all fat removed
115g/4oz cauliflower, boiled
2 medium courgettes, sliced and boiled

15ml/1 tablespoon mint sauce
175g/6oz potatoes, boiled
30ml/2 tablespoons gravy made without fat
1 medium apple

Or a keen cook's recipe **Lamb Olives and Vegetables**

115g/4oz raw leg of lamb or a very lean boneless chump chop, cut into two slices
5ml/1 level teaspoon butter
5ml/1 teaspoon honey
6 peach slices or 2 apricot halves, fresh or canned in low-calorie syrup or juice

15ml/1 level tablespoon finely chopped onion
25g/1oz fresh breadcrumbs
Pinch dried thyme
Salt and pepper
115g/4oz mushrooms
115g/4oz carrots, fresh or canned

Put the meat between two sheets of non-stick paper and beat until thin. Melt the butter and honey in a small pan and add the chopped peach, onion, breadcrumbs, thyme and seasoning. Divide the mixture between the meat slices and fold to enclose the stuffing. Tie with string. Wrap in foil and bake at 180°C, 350°F, gas mark 4, for 45 minutes. Remove the string and serve with mushrooms poached in stock or water and boiled carrots.

Or if you prefer to eat vegetarian **Vegetable Curry with Rice plus Orange**

50g/2oz raw brown long-grain rice
5ml/1 teaspoon vegetable oil
25g/1oz onion
50g/2oz cooking apple
5-10ml/1-2 level teaspoons curry powder
150ml/¼ pint water or vegetable stock
5ml/1 teaspoon tomato purée

5ml/1 teaspoon lemon juice
125g/4oz canned red kidney beans
125g/4oz frozen mixed vegetables
5ml/1 level teaspoon cornflour
Salt and pepper
1 medium orange

Cook the rice in boiling salted water for 30 minutes. Meanwhile, heat oil in a pan. Finely chop onion and peel, core and chop apple; cook gently in oil for 5 minutes without browning. Stir in the curry powder and cook for 2 minutes stirring all the time. Add the water or stock, bring to the boil, stirring, then add the tomato purée and lemon juice. Cover and simmer for 5 minutes. Add the drained kidney beans and thawed mixed vegetables. Bring to the boil, cover and simmer gently for 15 minutes. Blend cornflour with a little cold water and add to curry. Stir until thickened. Season to taste with salt and pepper. Arrange the rice on a warm serving dish and spoon the vegetable curry into the centre. Serve hot. Follow with orange.

Snack 1 ☐ *1 individual ice cream, any flavour*

Snack 2 ☐ *2 crispbreads*   *15ml/1 level tablespoon*
10ml/2 teaspoons yeast   *peanut butter*
   extract   *1 small banana*

☐ If you completed the day without cheating at all, tick here and move on to Day 8.

☐ If you cheated, do a 'Saintly Day' tomorrow (page 253) instead of the set menu.

☐ If you do not eat one meal or snack that you are allowed, tick this box and save up for a 'Naughty Day'. When you have two ticks saved, you can do any of the Thoroughly Naughty Day's Menus *instead* of your next day's diet.

Exercise Day 7

MORNING ☐ Repeat Exercise 1: 5 times

☐ Repeat Exercise 2: 5 times to right
5 times to left

☐ Repeat Exercise 3: 5 times circling left and right with right foot
5 times circling left and right with left foot

☐ Repeat Exercise 4: touch the floor 15 times

☐ Repeat Exercise 5: bend to the left and right. Do this 15 times.

Remember to put your alarm clock on slightly earlier each morning so that you do not have to rush through your exercises.

LUNCHTIME ☐ Walk for 11 minutes. Turn and return the same way in 9 minutes.

EVENING ☐ Run to the top of the stairs and down again twice. Jog on the spot for 3 minutes.

Or ☐ Jog for 8 minutes.

Bedtime Relaxer ☐

Beauty Day 7

Your hair is the most versatile part of your appearance. Nothing else can so instantly alter the way you look. But whether your style is simple or sophisticated, it's dependent for its good looks on your hair's condition.

Oily or dry?
This is fairly easy to judge. The happy norm is hair which stays bouncy for around 4 or 5 days before becoming oily and needing a shampoo.

Oily hair
Oily hair is essentially healthy hair. Oil from the sebaceous glands lubricates and protects hair, but too much overloads, 'flattens' and attracts dirt. An oily skin is usually partnered by oily hair. Washing hair every 2 or 3 days with a mild shampoo is the most effective way of removing excess oil. If hair is *very* oily, it may need to be washed every day. Do not use very hot water, though, because that can stimulate

oil glands into over-production and make the basic problem worse. Shampoo and rinse hair thoroughly, twice. If shampooing is delayed or hair is excessively oily, tip some cologne or bay rum on a piece of cotton wool and stroke it along partings combed through the hair, to revive it.

Dry hair

Dry hair and a dry scalp often go together. There's too little natural oil and, after washing, hair simply won't lie down. Conditioners can tame this 'flyaway' problem. Choose a conditionor especially formulated for dry hair and use a mild shampoo. For ultra-dry hair, a fine oil spray or a slick of almond oil rubbed over palms can be swished through hair when it's wet. Dry hair also needs protection from hairdryers and heated rollers.

Dandruff

Frequent shampooing may cope with very mild dandruff, but it usually pays to switch to anti-dandruff products. A powdering of flakes from a dry scalp may be mistaken for dandruff, but this can be dealt with using the warm oil treatment outlined below.

Today's special treatment

Try some lively scalp massage to relax tension and stimulate circulation. Sit comfortably. Drop your head forward. Begin at nape of the neck and massage with fingers in a spiral movement, spreading hands outwards to include the sides of the head and working towards forehead. Spend 3 or 4 minutes working up and over. Feel a glow? That proves the treatment is working, and it should give hair an extra bounce. Massage daily if hair is dry, every other day if it is oily.

For dry hair, dry scalp

Warm 2 tablespoons of almond oil by standing the bottle in hot water after loosening the cap. Massage warm oil into scalp and wrap a towel wrung out in hot water around head or heat with a hairdryer for 5 minutes. Allow oil to stay on scalp for 20 to 30 minutes, then shampoo hair thoroughly and follow with conditioner.

Cleanse, tone, moisturize

Cleanse, tone and moisturize your face in the morning and at night.

Goosepimples?

Lather goosepimply areas with a soft brush. Splash with cold water, pat dry and rub in cream or body lotion.

Do you love your body?

The woman who regards her own body with unalloyed satisfaction is very rare! This goes for young women, older women, plump women, slim women, even for top photographic models whose figures are quite undeniably their fortunes. Each of us, naturally, has an idea of how the 'perfect' body should look. But this whole issue of what is or is not acceptable or beautiful is largely determined by the society we happen to live in. For instance, at certain times in history women we would term fat have been regarded as the ideal. Think of Rubens' cushiony beauties! Or those thick-waisted, heavy-necked ladies so admired by the Pre-Raphaelite school of artists. Indeed, consider this item of anthropological research: of 26 widely-differing cultures from all over the world who happened to record their preference for a particular kind of female figure, only 5 cultures preferred slender silhouettes.

We are not for one moment suggesting that surplus weight is a good thing. We are, however, pointing out that the so-called 'perfect' body is a mainly arbitrary idea — and that we in the West could be said to be almost obsessed with a certain kind of slender shape. Led to some extent by the fashion industries, we tend to set an unduly high value on an unpadded clotheshorse of a shape; on long attenuated limbs, small bones and small waists. People are exposed to this idea of perfection almost every time they watch TV or open a magazine or newspaper. This is the type of body our society extols; the one that women have been conditioned to regard as the right kind to have.

Subconsciously many women feel that any departure from this (rare!) ideal is an imperfection. And they lament their height or lack of it, too-small or too-large bosoms, large thighs, wide hips, short legs and so on. Though there is no lack of evidence that many women who are considered very attractive, and indeed beautiful, are by no means physically perfect. Ordinary common sense and observation show that really there are remarkably few model faces and bodies around; and yet many women still feel that any deviation from the model ideal is somehow wrong. Now, if it makes a person regard herself as a failure, this is a matter for major concern.

Once past the super-sensitive teenage years, most of us learn to cope with the 'flaws' that nature handed out; we don't worry about them over much. But for some people, these imperfections become so important that they destroy self-confidence and act as a barrier to forming happy relationships, especially with the opposite sex.

Stretch marks are something which many women worry about. Complaints and queries come not only from women whose marks are the legacy of earlier weight problems, but also from women whose stretch marks result from childbearing. Many say they are so desperately unhappy about their unsightly marks that they cannot bear their bodies to be exposed. They fear to embark on a new relationship, or they may even unhappily withdraw from a familiar one. This is very sad. Stretch marks may not be desirable in themselves but in a sincerely loving relationship they are of little importance. You might say that for a woman to feel that stretch marks destroy her attractiveness is the equivalent of a man believing himself to be completely unlovable because he's started to go 'a bit thin on top'. Men love women and women love men not for their flawless looks but for themselves.

True, the confidence that goes with feeling happy about one's body tends to be a main attraction in the first place. We are all to some extent affected by attractive packaging! But if a man enjoys being in a woman's company and is genuinely attracted by her personality, then no physical imperfection — whether stretch marks or anything else — need mar the relationship. However, some women are so seriously disturbed by what they feel to be an insuperable physical flaw that they are afraid to become closely involved with another human being. They are often charming, useful and capable people, but their emotional lives have been blighted. Such a serious hang-up is often, in fact, unconsciously a mask for another kind of fear: the fear of getting too close to others. This may be the remnant of some deep emotional hurt that was perhaps inflicted in childhood or in an unhappy adult relationship. Such fear very often focuses on one imperfection — one part of the body that is felt to be hideous or unacceptable. Thus, stretch marks or too-small or too-large breasts or some other flaw will become a useful surface symbol for a much more profound depression and hidden fear.

This almost obsessive attitude to a physical imperfection — when brooding over it practically takes over a person's waking hours — needs very careful examination. Anyone who feels in this sort of state could find that it helps to talk to a sympathetic family doctor and, indeed, should perhaps ask to be referred to a psychotherapist, who is trained to help sort out people's underlying attitudes and bring them greater understanding of themselves and of their personal value. Usually, however, psychiatric or professional help is not needed. There are several very useful and very healing steps that you can take for yourself.

The first is to realize that, if you suffer to any degree from this kind of body hang-up, other people probably have not noticed your supposed defect — and, if they have, they are quite likely to regard it as an attractive part of the person you are. Other people will also have noticed your assets — all the nice, good things about your appearance which, in your concern with your problem, you have most probably entirely forgotten to consider or have even totally discounted. So, the second thing is to try to look at yourself as you really are, and make a mental list of all your good points. Maybe you have lovely hair, a creamy skin, or a particularly nice smile. You certainly have many more good things going for you than you have let yourself think, and they are as much part of you as the one imperfect part which gives you so much concern.

The way you present and hold yourself and the way you respond to other people are crucially important in relationships. They are all part of your 'body language': the secret subliminal signals we all send out to each other to say 'keep away' or 'I like myself and I like you'. The woman who is in some way ashamed of her body is liable, without realizing it, to keep sending out 'keep away' signals. She tends to dress in a nondescript, colourless way. Often, she will sit with her shoulders rounded and legs twisted. Her gestures may be unrelaxed and nervous. These are some of the signals that others subconsciously interpret as 'keep away', and, as a result, they will pay little attention to the person who sends them out.

Your body language and the way you look *can* be changed. Wearing becoming clothes and an air of confidence takes you more than halfway towards feeling attractive. Surplus weight in itself causes some of the most serious body hang-ups. Society says you have to be slim — and it's hard to think of any other section of society that suffers as much disapproval as the obese. It starts in childhood, right there in the school playground where the teasing of the fat child by other children may persuade her that she is 'unacceptable', 'ugly' and even a 'freak'. The girl who gains weight in adolescence can suffer greatly too. She usually has to cope with nicknames, teasing and taunting. She is the one who tends to be least wanted on a date, the girl who sits out at discos. And society in the main approves of this treatment. It has truly been said that the obese are

Disguising blemishes

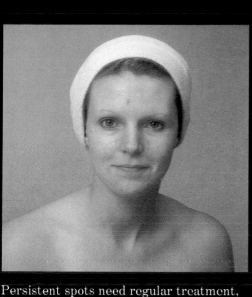 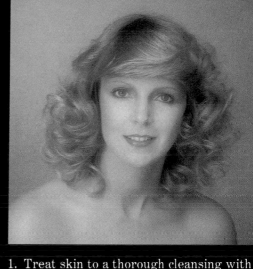

Persistent spots need regular treatment,
but on this page we show you how minor
blemishes can be successfully camouflaged.
Pat Watkinson, before and after,
also had deep-set eyes and over-plucked
brows.

1. Treat skin to a thorough cleansing with
a medicated cleanser or soap and water
before beginning your make-up. Dab spots
with diluted antiseptic and allow it to dry.
2. Blot out spots with a medicated
treatment stick. Select a shade nearest to
your skin tone or one that's slightly lighter
Take care to blend it into your skin around
the spots to avoid hard edges.
3. Stroke on a light tinted fluid foundation
which matches your natural skin shade. Go
gently over the spotty areas. Then press
loose powder all over your face. Brush off
surplus, taking extra care where spots are
camouflaged.
4. Eye shadow was softly applied to the
outer corners of Pat's eyes and her lids
highlighted. Her brows were re-shaped and
softened with tiny hair-like strokes in
charcoal-grey eyebrow pencil.
5. Pat's make-up was completed with a
soft-toned lip colour.

Achieving a natural look

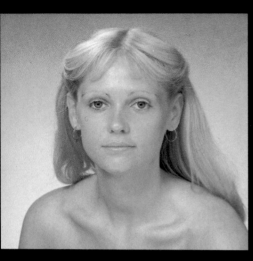

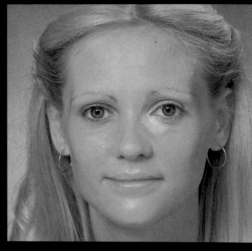

Shaun Williams lost a hefty 5st and felt this called for a fresh approach to an excitingly slimmer face. Fair, fragile colouring only requires the softest make-up. Hard lines are taboo — no heavy eyelining or sharp, over-plucked brows. Here is Shaun unadorned and we show how we achieved her transformation.

1. First cover face with a fluid foundation that matches your skin tone. Blot out any dingy shadows round the eye with a pale covering cream. Shaun painted it right round her whole eye area with a small brush, but you could use light finger strokes.

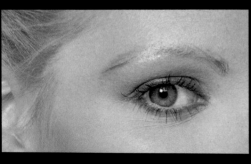

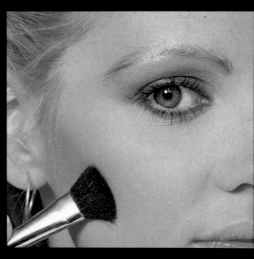

2. Keep brows feathery and not too fine. Sketch light, feathery strokes with a grey-brown eye pencil — beware of using a gingery colour though! Use this pencil to define eyes, blurring the colour carefully with a small brush. Highlight brow bone with a subtle pearly highlighter.

3. Go for soft beigey-coral blusher. Curve

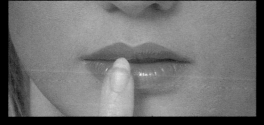

4. Colour lips softly: creamy peach, apricot or coral. Choose a glossy lipstick for a specially soft effect or add a topping of lip gloss or petroleum jelly.

5. See, it works. Shaun has camouflaged problem areas without looking over made-up.

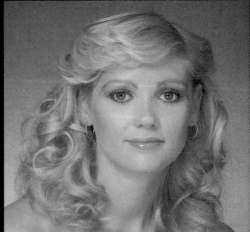

Making up a round face

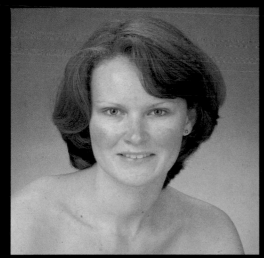

Brush off the surplus powder in a downward direction using cotton wool or a powder brush.

3. Play up your eyes. Make them larger and more lustrous with highlighter on lids, brush-blended into golden brown above. Brush golden brown shadow upwards and outwards to brows. Draw a fine pencil line at outer corners of eyes.

4. Use blusher to shape and disguise. Choose the powder block type and brush it low on outer cheeks to emphasize cheekbones. Smile to create cheek 'cushions' and brush inwards beneath them.

5. Keep mouth colour soft but warm-toned. Key it to blusher shade. Add gloss if, like Nicci, you have a pretty mouth.

If, like Nicci Wilson above, you have shed surplus weight but found that your face was still basically a bit too round in shape, make-up can help. Above is Nicci before our make-up artist got to work. On the right is Nicci after her face had been shaped up to a new kind of loveliness. Here's how you can do the same.

1. Apply a skin-toning foundation over your face. Opt for a creamy beige if, like Nicci, you are bothered by high colour. A make-up stick, more opaque than fluid bases, provides good cover.

2. Press on fine, loose translucent powder.

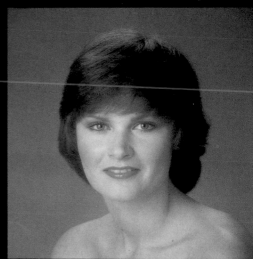

Making up a square face

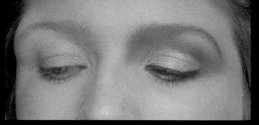

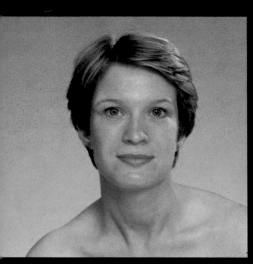

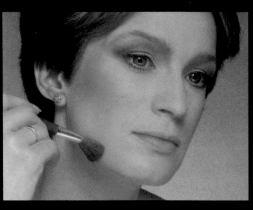

3. Emphasize your eyes with sheeny highlighter on lids. Stroke it over eye shading to blend the colours and soften.

Paulyne Kelly lost 3½ stone and wanted a new look for her face. Bare-faced, above, Paulyne has a square jawline and a wide nose bridge which overshadows her attractive blue eyes.

1. Smooth on a tinted foundation. Press on fine, loose translucent powder. Brush off any surplus with cotton wool or a powder brush.

2. Apply eye shadow at outer eye. Extend colour inwards if, like Paulyne, you wish to minimize a broad nose bridge. Tilt the shading upwards at outer eye. This is a good trick for 'knocking back' a prominent brow bone; it works well, too, for an older face which needs a lift.

4. Curve blusher beneath cheekbones to create an illusion of elegant, high-boned cheeks. Shade low on chin either side of jawline to round off the corners and minimize squareness.

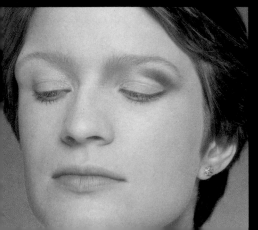

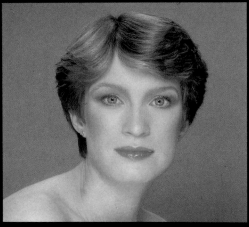

5. To complete your make-up, use a strong lip colour but avoid a very bright or dark lipstick or your mouth will dominate your face. Here is Paulyne with her new look, which highlights her good points and draws attention away from her problem areas.

'sanctioned victims'. Though accepted rules of polite
behaviour strongly forbid us to insult other people for any
physical peculiarity they may have, the rule tends to relax
where fat people are concerned, leaving them very
vulnerable. Many obese women know the embarrassment of
having 'Fatty' shouted at them from passing cars. They are
used to friends, and even total strangers, making such
personal remarks as: 'You know, you could be quite nice-
looking if you lost a couple of stones.' What other disability
calls forth such gratuitous insults and advice? But, because
she is conditioned by today's standards of beauty, the
overweight woman may grow to believe that unkindness
and hostility are simply her due, because she has 'sinned' in
not conforming to the contemporary ideal of feminine
shapeliness.

It is this low self-esteem that makes it so difficult for
many women to keep to a diet and to lose weight.
Somewhere deep down, they feel they are not only
unlovable now because they are fat but are also
permanently unlovable because they 'deserve' to be
rejected. This fundamental feeling of unworthiness and
very low self-regard has to be explored — and then
exploded! While it remains, it leads to many difficulties.
One is that a woman who believes she is unacceptable will
tend to place unrealistic demands on herself in terms of a
'perfect' diet. The diet she plans will be so punishing that
she will just be unable to stick with it for very long. The
moment she breaks it and breaks out — which, being
human, she will — back will come the feelings of
unworthiness to destroy any faith in her ability to succeed.
Another very real problem is that she will often tend to
believe that all her troubles arise because she is
overweight. The expectation is: 'When I'm slim, my sex life
will pick up, my marriage will be happy again, everything
will be marvellous.'

This won't necessarily be true, alas. An improvement in
the 'packaging' can give a great positive boost to the
personality inside — but it is still basically the same
personality, with all its old strengths and weaknesses. And
so the time to explore what is wrong with a relationship or
with your life is always *now*. It is easy to blame obesity —
or any other physical flaw — as the main reason why a
relationship has gone sour. Obesity is particularly easy to
blame because of its conditioned association with ugliness,
gluttony and sin . . . But if there is something wrong with
your life or the way you feel about yourself, it is far more
productive to learn to start viewing yourself with more

understanding and kindness. Much unhappiness is caused by surplus weight — but happiness and confidence need not depend on being slim, and there is no reason why they should not be yours now.

Week 2

☐☐ Weigh yourself and write in your weight here

☐☐ Now check the chart on page 7 and write in your ideal weight here

☐☐ Write in the amount you have to lose here

Now tick one of these boxes, and this is your menu plan for this week

☐ If you have under 1st to lose, you can have breakfast/supper, a light meal and a main meal each day.

☐ If you have between 1st and 3st to lose, you can have breakfast/supper, a light meal, a main meal and one snack.

☐ If you have over 3st to lose, you can have breakfast/supper, a light meal, a main meal and two snacks.

Shopping Checklist Day 8

Choose your meals, then write in by each relevant item the amount you require.

Amount required	Amount required	Amount required
Fruit and Vegetables	Low-fat raspberry	Marmalade or jam
Carrots	yogurt	Oil-free French
Mushrooms	Skimmed milk	dressing
Onion	**Grocery**	Oregano or thyme
Tomato	Dried apricots	Salt and pepper
Banana	Baked beans in	Sherry
Kiwi fruit	tomato sauce	Stock cube
Orange	Biscuits, digestive,	Tomato purée
Pear	ginger snap or	Vegetable oil
Strawberries	muesli	Yeast extract
Frozen foods	Bran breakfast cereal	
Broad beans	Canned tomatoes	
Broccoli	Chocolate flavour	
Carrots	sauce	
Peas	Cream crackers or	
Runner beans	water biscuits	
Strawberries	Hazelnuts	
Sweetcorn	Low-calorie	
Meat, Poultry and Fish	packet soup	
Chipolata sausage	Rice	
Kidneys	Textured vegetable	
Streaky bacon	protein mince	
Dairy Produce/Eggs	Wholemeal bread	
Camembert cheese	Wholewheat spaghetti	
Eggs	**Store cupboard**	
Low-fat spread	Cornflour	

Diet Day 8

☐ 275ml/½ pint skimmed milk or reconstituted low-fat powdered milk

BREAKFAST/SUPPER MEAL

Either ☐ 2 eggs, size 3; 15ml/1 tablespoon skimmed milk; 1 tomato
Scramble eggs with milk. Serve with tomato grilled without fat.

Or ☐ 25g/1oz any bran breakfast cereal; 75ml/5 tablespoons skimmed milk; 2 dried apricots, chopped

Or ☐ 2 small slices wholemeal bread, 25g/1oz each, toasted; 10ml/2 level teaspoons low-fat spread; 10ml/2 level teaspoons marmalade or jam

LIGHT MEAL

Either to eat at home
Baked Beans, Tomato and Bacon plus Biscuits
☐

150g/5.3oz can baked beans	2 tomatoes
2 rashers streaky bacon	2 small digestive biscuits

Heat beans and serve with well-grilled bacon and tomatoes grilled without fat. Follow with biscuits.

Or to take to work
Soup, Bean and Bacon Salad plus Biscuits
☐

1 sachet low-calorie instant soup, any flavour	50g/2oz sweetcorn, frozen or canned
2 rashers streaky bacon	25g/1oz onion
50g/2oz broad beans, frozen	15ml/1 level tablespoon oil-free French dressing
50g/2oz runner beans, frozen	2 ginger snap biscuits

Mix soup with boiling water at work or take to work in a flask. Well grill bacon and chop. Boil beans and frozen sweetcorn, drain and allow to cool. Mix beans and sweetcorn with finely chopped onion, bacon and dressing. Take to work in a container. Finish meal with biscuits.

Or if you prefer to eat vegetarian
Bean and Tomato Soup plus Biscuits
☐

25g/1oz onion	150g/5.3oz can baked beans in tomato sauce
1 tomato	
5ml/1 teaspoon vegetable oil	1.25ml/¼ teaspoon yeast extract
225ml/8floz vegetable stock or water	Salt and pepper
	2 muesli biscuits

69

Stir-fry chopped onion and tomato in oil in a non-stick pan for 2 minutes. Add vegetable stock or water, bring to the boil, cover and simmer for 5 minutes. Stir in the baked beans and yeast extract. Purée the soup in a blender or sieve, then reheat. Season to taste with salt and pepper. Follow with biscuits.

MAIN MEAL

Either a quick meal **Kidney, Rice and Vegetables plus Chocolate Banana**

2 lamb's kidneys
30ml/2 level tablespoons raw rice
50g/2oz peas
75g/3oz carrots

1 small banana
15ml/1 tablespoon chocolate-flavour sauce
5ml/1 level teaspoon chopped hazelnuts

Halve, core and grill kidneys. Boil rice, peas and diced carrots and serve with kidneys. Peel and slice banana and serve topped with chocolate sauce and sprinkle with toasted hazelnuts.

Or a keen cook's recipe **Kidneys in Sherry Sauce, Rice and Vegetables**

2 lamb's kidneys
1 small onion
5ml/1 level teaspoon cornflour
60ml/4 tablespoons stock made with ¼ stock cube
25g/1oz button mushrooms
5ml/1 level teaspoon tomato purée

Salt and pepper
1 pork chipolata sausage
10ml/2 teaspoons sherry
30ml/2 level tablespoons raw rice
150g/5oz runner beans or broccoli
1 medium orange

Halve and core the kidneys, thinly slice the onion. Mix cornflour with stock until smooth; heat, stirring, until boiling. Reduce heat and add kidneys, onion, mushrooms, tomato purée and seasoning. Simmer for about 20 minutes, adding more water if necessary. Meanwhile, grill sausage well and cut in 4. Add to the kidneys together with the sherry. Boil the rice and greens and serve with kidneys. Follow with the orange.

Or if you prefer to eat vegetarian **Spaghetti with Vegetable Bolognese plus Pear**

25g/1oz textured vegetable protein mince dry
225g/8oz canned tomatoes
1 small onion
15ml/1 level tablespoon tomato purée
2.5ml/½ level teaspoon yeast extract

Pinch dried oregano or thyme
50g/2oz wholewheat spaghetti
1 medium pear

Reconstitute the textured vegetable protein mince with water as directed. Roughly chop canned tomatoes and place in a pan with peeled and chopped onion, vegetable mince, tomato purée, yeast extract and herbs. Bring to the boil, stirring. Reduce heat, cover and simmer for 15-20 minutes. Meanwhile cook the spaghetti in boiling salted water for 12 minutes; drain and serve with vegetable bolognese. Follow with the pear.

Snack 1 ☐ *1 small carton low-fat raspberry yogurt*   *115g/4oz strawberries, fresh or frozen*
1 kiwi fruit or pear
Mix fruit with yogurt or eat separately.

Snack 2 ☐ *3 cream crackers or large water biscuits*   *1 individual portion Camembert cheese, 35g/1¼oz*

☐ If you completed the day without cheating at all, tick here and move on to Day 9.

☐ If you cheated, do a 'Saintly Day' tomorrow (page 253) instead of the set menu.

☐ If you do not eat one meal or snack that you are allowed, tick this box and save up for a 'Naughty Day'. When you have two ticks saved, you can do any of the Thoroughly Naughty Day's Menus *instead* of your next day's diet.

Exercise Day 8

MORNING ☐ Repeat Exercise 1: 5 times

☐ Repeat Exercise 2: 5 times to right
5 times to left

☐ Repeat Exercise 3: 5 times circling left and right with right foot
5 times circling left and right with left foot

Repeat Exercise 4: touch the floor 15 times

Repeat Exercise 5: bend to the left and right 15 times

Exercise 6   Stand with feet apart and relax forward from waist, bending knees slightly. Link fingers loosely together and circle arms to left, above head and down to right, finishing in original position. Circle to left 4 more times. Then circle to right 5 times.

LUNCHTIME   Walk for 12 minutes. Turn and return the same way in 10 minutes.

EVENING   Run to the top of the stairs and down again twice. Jog on the spot or around the house or garden for 4 minutes.

Or   Jog for 9 minutes.

Bedtime Relaxer

Beauty Shopping List Week 2

The number of items you will require depends on your skin type and problems. Check through the week's treatments and write down the products you need to purchase.

Almond oil	Flour	Powdered milk
Baby oil	Hand lotion	Pumice stone
Bleaching cream	Honey	Razor
Body lotion	Lemon juice	Salt
Buffing paste	Manicure stick	10-volume peroxide
Cleanser	Medicated soap	Toner
Cuticle cream	Medicated talc	Tweezers
Depilatory cream	Moisturizer	Waterproof emery
Depilatory wax	Nail clippers or	paper
Egg yolk	scissors	Yogurt
Emery board	Nail polish	
Fat	Nail polish remover	

Beauty Day 8

Look around. See what separates the young from the old. Not just the obvious signs. There are many people with grey hair and wrinkles who manage to stay young and vital. Watch how people *move*. The young are usually light on their feet, straight-backed, movements free, fluid and speedy — unless they are hampered by being overweight. But watch people who shamble along, heads bent, shoulders and backs rounded. They appear older, whatever their age. Posture says a lot about people. Round shoulders can be a sign of painful feet. Help for those can be found on page 80,

Day 9. Or a drooping head usually says: 'I'm bored/
miserable/shy/lack confidence.' A shuffle is plainly not
pretty. It's often a shock to be confronted by the truth at
unexpected moments, reflected in a shop window or
exposed in a photograph; it's so easy to cheat in front of a
looking-glass.

Try an instant 'before and after' exercise on yourself.
Stand before a full-length looking-glass. Drop your head,
hunch your shoulders, let your stomach sag. Then
straighten up: shoulders back but relaxed, head up, neck
swan-like, stomach in, seat tucked in but without strain.
Obvious which looks more attractive, isn't it?

Today's special treatment

Test your stance Stand with your back to the
wall. Head, shoulders,
bottom and heels should
touch without strain. An
ache in your shoulders could
indicate that they need
loosening up. This will come
if you continue your daily
exercises.

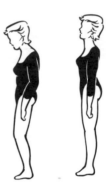

Walk gracefully Balance a book on your head and move around the room.
It's an old idea but it still has value. Can you feel your body
straightening? *That's* the way you should always walk.
Look straight ahead, not down at your feet, and glide along
like the models do. If you have the chance, attend a fashion
show and see how the professionals walk.

Sit serenely Lower your body *lightly* into a chair. Young actors playing
the part of someone older are taught to 'bottom drop': they
have to learn how it feels to sit stiffly and heavily. To sit
the right way, place your bottom well back in the chair, legs
together and slanting sideways from knees. Cross one ankle
over the other if that makes you feel more comfortable.
Avoid crossing legs at the knees as this can impede
circulation. Clasp hands loosely in your lap. Make yourself
conscious of holding your hands together: a great help if
you are feeling nervous.

Practise
standing tall Stand with your feet together. Lift up your toes, then put
them back on the floor stretching them forwards. Check
that you are standing evenly on both feet, straighten legs,

pulling up from the ankle. Lift shoulders up towards the ears: then, moving them back, allow them to fall in a relaxed position. Now look ahead and work at stretching your whole body upwards. Keep your feet flat on the floor and your chin tucked in. Feel yourself growing taller and your spine straightening out.

Bend beautifully

If you have to lift something from the floor, bend knees and lower body into a semi-sitting position. It makes a prettier shape than bending over with knees stiff — and it is less of a strain on the spine. Keep your thinking supple. Be aware of your every move, and eventually your new habits will become natural and spontaneous. Why not ask family or friends to remind you when they catch you slouching? Discreetly, of course!

Cleanse, tone, moisturize

Cleanse, tone and moisturize your face in the morning and at night.

Hair livener

Massage scalp, see page 61, Day 7, but omit oil.

Blackheads?

Repeat steam treatment from page 42, Day 4.

Shopping Checklist Day 9

Choose your meals, then write in by each relevant item the amount you require.

Amount required	Amount required	Amount required
Fruit and Vegetables	**Dairy Produce/Eggs**	**Store cupboard**
Brussels sprouts	Butter	Golden syrup
Cauliflower	Cottage cheese	Low-calorie salad
Chicory or lettuce	Edam or Tendale	dressing
Cucumber	cheese	Mustard pickle
Green pepper	Eggs	or sweet pickle
Lettuce	Low-fat natural yogurt	Oil-free French
Mushrooms	Low-fat spread	dressing
Onion	Skimmed milk	Salt and pepper
Potato	**Grocery**	Tarragon
Radishes	Bran breakfast cereal	Tomato purée
Tomatoes	Canned butter beans	White wine
Watercress	Canned tomatoes	
Apricot	Corn snacks	
Banana	Creamed rice	
Cooking apple	Fruit salad or	
Peach	fruit cocktail in	
Frozen foods	low-calorie syrup	
Brussels sprouts	Pasta shells	
Cauliflower	Peaches or apricots,	
Individual chicken and	canned in low-calorie	
mushroom casserole	syrup or juice	
Meat, Poultry and Fish	Pitta bread	
Chicken breast	Raisins or	
Streaky bacon	sultanas	
	Wholemeal bread	

Diet Day 9

275ml/½ pint skimmed milk or reconstituted low-fat powdered milk

BREAKFAST/SUPPER MEAL

Either
1 slice wholemeal bread, 40g/1½oz; 1 egg, size 3; 5ml/1 level teaspoon low-fat spread
Dip bread in beaten egg and fry in non-stick pan greased with low-fat spread.

Or
25g/1oz any bran breakfast cereal; 75ml/5 tablespoons skimmed milk (extra to allowance); 30ml/2 level tablespoons raisins or sultanas

Or
2 tomatoes, grilled without fat; 2 rashers streaky bacon, well grilled; 1 small slice wholemeal bread, 25g/1oz

LIGHT MEAL

Either to eat at home
Baked Potato and Salad

175g/6oz potato
25g/1oz Edam or Tendale cheese
Lettuce

Cucumber
Watercress
15ml/1 tablespoon oil-free French dressing

Scrub the potato and bake at 200°C/400°F, gas mark 6, for 1 hour. Halve potato and top with grated Edam or Tendale cheese. Grill until cheese bubbles. Serve potato with green salad made with lettuce, cucumber, watercress and dressing.

Or to take to work
Cheese and Salad Pitta

1 pitta bread or 2 large slices wholemeal bread, 40g/1½oz each
Cucumber
Radishes
Watercress
4 chicory leaves or lettuce

15ml/1 level tablespoon mustard pickle or sweet pickle
25g/1oz Edam or Tendale cheese
2 tomatoes

Open up pitta bread to form a pocket. Dice cucumber, slice a few radishes, chop a few sprigs of watercress and thinly slice chicory. Use to fill pitta pocket mixed with pickle and grated cheese. Take tomatoes to eat with pitta. If you are using bread slices, spread them with pickle and make into a sandwich with cheese and salad.

*Either a
quick recipe*
**Chicken and
Mushroom
Casserole plus
Peach and Rice**

1 individual frozen chicken
  and mushroom casserole
115g/4oz Brussels sprouts
115g/4oz cauliflower

175g/6oz can creamed rice
1 peach or apricot, fresh or
  canned in low-calorie syrup
  or juice

Cook chicken and mushroom casserole as instructed on
packet and serve with boiled sprouts and cauliflower. Heat
rice and mix with sliced peach or apricot.

---

*Or a keen
cook's recipe*
**Stuffed Chicken
Breast and
Vegetables
plus
Baked Apple**

115g/4oz boned chicken
  breast
5ml/1 level teaspoon butter
25g/1oz onion
50g/2oz mushrooms
Salt and pepper
Small pinch tarragon
15ml/1 level tablespoon fresh
  breadcrumbs

15ml/1 tablespoon natural
  yogurt
30ml/2 level tablespoons
  stock or white wine
115g/4oz Brussels sprouts
115g/4oz cauliflower
150g/5oz cooking apple
15ml/1 level tablespoon
  golden syrup

Remove skin from the chicken and cut the breast two-thirds
of the way through lengthways. Place between 2 pieces
of non-stick paper and beat until about twice the size. Put
the butter, finely chopped onion and thinly sliced mushrooms
in a small pan and heat gently for 5 minutes. Add seasoning,
breadcrumbs and yogurt. Mix thoroughly. Spread the filling
on the chicken and fold over. Secure with cocktail sticks.
Place on a sheet of aluminium foil, pour over stock or wine
and fold the foil to make a loose but secure package. Bake at
180°C/350°F gas mark 4, for about 1 hour. Serve with
boiled sprouts and cauliflower. Core apple and cut the skin
around the middle. Stand apple in an ovenproof dish and
spoon the golden syrup into the centre cavity. Place 30ml/2
tablespoons water in the dish and bake with chicken for last
30 minutes.

---

*Or if you
prefer to eat
vegetarian*
**Butter Bean
Pie plus
Banana**

1 small onion
Half a 200g/7oz can tomatoes
½ green pepper
Half a 213g/7½oz can butter
  beans
15ml/1 level tablespoon
  tomato purée

Salt and pepper
1 egg, size 3
115g/4oz cottage cheese
1 medium banana

Cook chopped onion in a little juice from tomatoes, then add
chopped tomatoes and pepper. Cook for 2 minutes. Mix
drained butter beans with tomato purée and put into a
small casserole dish. Add onion, tomatoes and pepper.
Season. Beat egg into cottage cheese and spread over

beans. Bake at 180°C/350°F, gas mark 4, for 30 minutes, until topping is set and golden brown. Follow with the banana.

Snack 1 ☐ *113g/4oz carton cottage cheese with chives, with onion and peppers or with pineapple*   *1 small packet corn snacks, any flavour*

Snack 2 ☐ *227g/8oz can fruit salad or fruit cocktail in low-calorie syrup*   *30ml/2 tablespoons low-fat natural yogurt*

25g/1oz pasta shells   *15ml/1 tablespoon low-calorie salad dressing*

Drain fruit. Boil pasta, drain and mix with fruit. Mix the yogurt with salad dressing and add to fruit and pasta.

☐ If you completed the day without cheating at all, tick here and move on to Day 10.

☐ If you cheated, do a 'Saintly Day' tomorrow (page 253) instead of the set menu.

☐ If you do not eat one meal or snack that you are allowed, tick this box and save up for a 'Naughty Day'. When you have two ticks saved, you can do any of the Thoroughly Naughty Day's Menus *instead* of your next day's diet.

Exercise Day 9

MORNING ☐ Repeat Exercise 1: 5 times

☐ Repeat Exercise 2: 5 times to right
5 times to left

☐ Repeat Exercise 3: 5 times circling left and right with right foot
5 times circling left and right with left foot

☐ Repeat Exercise 4: touch the floor 15 times

☐ Repeat Exercise 5: bend to the left and right 15 times

☐ Repeat Exercise 6: circle to left 10 times
circle to right 10 times
Straighten your legs as you stretch upwards, keeping your feet flat on the floor. Stretch out as far as you can as you circle to the left and right.

LUNCHTIME ☐ Walk for 13 minutes. Turn and return the same way in 11 minutes.

EVENING ☐ Run to the top of the stairs and down again 3 times. Jog for 5 minutes.

Or ☐ Jog for 10 minutes.

Bedtime Relaxer ☐

Beauty Day 9

Feet should get a standing ovation for the wonderful way they support our weight. Too often they get forgotten until they begin to ache. Their structure is so intricately balanced that, if one of the many tiny bones gets out of balance, the whole foot suffers.

Many foot faults can be avoided, and bad shoes are mostly to blame. This doesn't necessarily mean that high heels are completely banned, though they do throw weight forward, putting unnatural pressure on the instep and the ball of the foot. So it makes sense to alternate with a lower heel now and again. A narrow pinching shoe can do more harm, squashing the large toe joint so that ultimately it becomes inflamed and thickens, and that's how bunions are born. Badly-fitting shoes can build up callouses, thick hard skin which forms on soles and heels, and corns appear at pressure points — they are simply the poor foot's way of protecting itself. Troubles of this kind should be taken to a chiropodist. Afterwards, keep callouses under control by rubbing with a pumice stone or waterproof emery paper when the skin is soft from bathing. Be a wise shoe shopper. Try on shoes late in the day, because most feet tend to swell slightly by the afternoon. The sales assistant may try to persuade you that a too-tight shoe will loosen with wear. It may, but meanwhile you have to live with the discomfort.

Today's special treatment

Take a good look at your feet. If you have callouses, corns or a build-up of hard skin, make an appointment with a chiropodist. Once your feet are in better condition, keep them in good shape by regularly following the treatment outlined below. Even if you have no particular feet problems, you should try this treatment to help stop hard skin forming and to smarten up nails.

1. Soak feet in soapy water for 10 minutes. Rub away hard skin with a pumice stone or waterproof emery paper.

2. Dry feet and cut nails straight across with clippers or small scissors. Round off sharp corners, but do not cut your nail too short as this can encourage an ingrowing toe nail.

3. Massage in cuticle cream and gently ease round the cuticle with a manicure stick wrapped in cotton wool. Ease stick around the sides of large toe nails to free any build-up of skin. Scrape lightly behind tops of nails.

4. Sponge feet to remove any debris and dry thoroughly.

5. Apply polish as for fingernails (see page 132, Day 16) or buff nails to make them shine. Rubbing in almond oil or a paste polish will give them a rosy hue.

6. Massage feet with hand lotion to leave them soft and silky. Stroke from toes to ankle on top of foot. Place fingers under feet, thumbs above, and pull along foot and up over heel.

7. Now sit with your feet raised, legs resting on a chair, stool or low table for a minimum of 10 minutes.

Cleanse, tone, moisturize

Cleanse, tone and moisturize your face in the morning and at night.

Body massage

Repeat the body massage from page 29, Day 2 before bed.

Hair livener

For dry hair only: massage scalp, see page 61, Day 7, but omit oil.

Shopping Checklist Day 10

Choose your meals, then write in by each relevant item the amount you require.

Amount required	Amount required	Amount required
Fruit and Vegetables	Edam or Tendale	Mixed herbs
Broad beans	cheese	Oil-free French
Carrots	Eggs	dressing
Cucumber	Low-fat spread	Salt and pepper
Green pepper	Skimmed milk	Stock cube
Onion	**Grocery**	Tomato purée
Parsley	Bran breakfast cereal	
Tomatoes	Canned broad beans	
Apple	Canned peeled	
Pear	tomatoes	
Frozen foods	Crispbreads	
Broad beans	Crisps	
Fish fingers	Muesli bar	
Fruit water ice	Peaches or apricots,	
or sorbet	canned in low-calorie	
Peas	syrup or juice	
Shepherd's pie	Pears in low-	
Sweetcorn	calorie syrup or	
Vanilla ice cream	water	
Meat, Poultry and Fish	Raisins	
Chipolata sausages	Red kidney beans	
Very lean	Rice	
minced beef	Sweetcorn, canned	
Dairy Produce/Eggs	Wholemeal bread	
Cheddar cheese	**Store cupboard**	
Cottage cheese	Cornflour	

Diet Day 10

☐ 275ml/½ pint skimmed milk or reconstituted low-fat powdered milk

BREAKFAST/SUPPER MEAL

Either ☐ 2 tomatoes, grilled without fat, or half a 227g/8oz can tomatoes; 2 chipolata sausages, well grilled; 1 small slice wholemeal bread, 25g/1oz

Or ☐ 1 egg, size 3, boiled; 1 slice wholemeal bread, 25g/1oz; 5ml/1 level teaspoon low-fat spread

Or ☐ 25g/1oz any bran breakfast cereal; 75ml/5 tablespoons skimmed milk; 15ml/1 level tablespoon raisins or 2 peaches or apricots canned in low-calorie syrup or juice

LIGHT MEAL

Either to eat at home
Fish Fingers and Salad plus Ice Cream

☐ 3 fish fingers / 15ml/1 tablespoon oil-free
Cucumber and onion / French dressing
2 tomatoes / 50g/2oz vanilla ice cream
Grill fish fingers without fat and serve with a salad of cucumber, onion and tomatoes sprinkled with dressing. Follow with ice cream.

Or to take to work
Pear and Cottage Cheese Salad

☐ 1 can pears in low-calorie syrup or water / 2 tomatoes, quartered
2 crispbreads
113g/4oz carton cottage cheese
Drain pears and put them at the bottom of a plastic container or large empty cottage cheese carton. Pile cottage cheese in the centre. Arrange quartered tomatoes around the sides. Take crispbreads to work separately and eat with salad. Or eat crispbreads with cottage cheese and tomatoes and follow with pears.

MAIN MEAL

Either a quick recipe
Shepherd's Pie plus Apple

☐ 227g/8oz frozen shepherd's pie / 115g/4oz broad beans
1 medium apple
115g/4oz carrots

Cook shepherd's pie as instructed on packet. Boil carrots and broad beans. Follow with apple.

Or a keen cook's recipe **Stuffed Peppers with Tomato Sauce and Rice plus Pear**

1 green pepper
75g/3oz very lean minced beef
1 small onion
Pinch mixed herbs
10ml/2 level teaspoons tomato purée
Salt and pepper
30ml/2 tablespoons stock made with ¼ stock cube

200g/7oz can peeled tomatoes
10ml/2 level teaspoons cornflour
45ml/3 level tablespoons raw long-grain rice
115g/4oz frozen peas
1 medium pear

Cut stalk end from pepper and retain. Scoop out and discard seeds. Put meat in a non-stick pan and brown. Drain off any fat. Add finely chopped onion, herbs, tomato purée, seasoning and stock, cover and simmer for 10 minutes. Push mixture into pepper and replace top. Put the stuffed pepper into a small ovenproof dish. To make the sauce, strain the tomato juice into a small saucepan and heat. Mix cornflour with a little cold water until smooth. Pour into tomato juice, stirring. Add the tomatoes and heat through, stirring. Season to taste. Pour tomato sauce over the pepper and bake at 190°C/375°F, gas mark 5, for 30 minutes. Boil rice and peas. Mix together and serve with stuffed pepper. Follow with pear.

Or if you prefer to eat vegetarian **Bean and Sweetcorn Salad plus Sorbet**

50g/2oz red kidney beans, canned
50g/2oz broad beans, frozen or canned
115g/4oz sweetcorn, frozen or canned
1 small onion

30ml/2 tablespoons oil-free French dressing
25g/1oz Edam or Tendale cheese
Fresh parsley
50g/2oz portion fruit water ice or sorbet, any flavour

Rinse and drain kidney beans. Boil the frozen broad beans and sweetcorn and drain. Cut onion into rings. Mix vegetables with dressing. Sprinkle grated Edam or Tendale cheese and chopped parsley on top. Follow with water ice or sorbet.

Snack 1

1 small packet crisps

25g/1oz Cheddar cheese

Snack 2

1 muesli bar

☐ If you completed the day without cheating at all, tick here and move on to Day 11.

☐ If you cheated, do a 'Saintly Day' tomorrow (page 253) instead of the set menu.

☐ If you do not eat one meal or snack that you are allowed, tick this box and save up for a 'Naughty Day'. When you have two ticks saved, you can do any of the Thoroughly Naughty Day's Menus *instead* of your next day's diet.

Exercise Day 10

MORNING ☐ Repeat Exercise 1: 5 times

☐ Repeat Exercise 2: 5 times to right
5 times to left

☐ Repeat Exercise 3: 5 times circling left and right with right foot
5 times circling left and right with left foot

☐ Repeat Exercise 4: touch the floor 15 times

☐ Repeat Exercise 5: bend to the left and right 15 times

☐ Repeat Exercise 6: circle to the left 15 times
circle to the right 15 times

LUNCHTIME ☐ Walk for 14 minutes. Turn and return the same way in 12 minutes.

EVENING ☐ Run to the top of the stairs and down again 3 times. Jog for 6 minutes.

Or ☐ Jog for 11 minutes.

Bedtime Relaxer ☐

Beauty Day 10

Body hair is naturally present everywhere except on the palms and on the soles of feet. It's mostly not a beauty bother, except when it shows up in inconvenient places. Unwanted hair ranges from a downy growth on the upper lip to thick stragglers on the chin and cheeks, and a thicker growth on arms and legs; noticeable hair in the nipple area is also quite a common problem. So, with today's skimpy swimsuits, is pubic hair that strays beyond bikini limits.

There are several ways of removing hair and many women use one or other of the methods quite regularly. Hair reappears unless the root is destroyed and this is the aim of electrolysis, which conveys a gentle electrical impulse through a needle inserted into the hair follicle. It's a treatment used most frequently for coping with facial hair and requires the expertise of a fully-trained operator. It can be a lengthy and expensive business — so it's advisable to ask for an estimate of cost before embarking on it.

Home treatment can work well to control excess hair. A downy growth can be lightened, and there are several effective bleaching creams on the market. Check first if they are for facial use or for lightening hair growth on arms and legs. Or mix a home-made bleach with 5 drops of household ammonia and 2 tablespoons of 20-volume peroxide. Dab it on with cotton wool but don't use near the eyes. Rinse off with cool water after 7-10 minutes. Repeat the treatment, but not for at least another 48 hours, until hair lightens.

Depilatory Cream
Hair can be removed with a depilatory cream and this is effective for obstinate facial hair, stray hairs over stomach and under-arm or leg growth. Regrowth needs treating within a week or two.

Depilatory waxes
These remove hair for a longer period because they pluck it from nearer the root. The wax is normally applied in strips and ripped off carefully when it hardens.

Shaving
This is sometimes thought to encourage hair growth but that's because the hair grows back blunted and feels prickly. It's quicker to shave but hair returns sooner than

with other methods because you don't remove any hair below the surface of the skin. If you decide on shaving, confine it to under arms and legs.

Tweezering
This is not just for eyebrows. Tweezers can be used to remove stragglers on face and around nipples. Which tweezers to choose? See page 98, Day 12.

Superfluous hair is a nuisance but nothing worse. With regular care it can be kept under control. It's mainly a matter of treating regrowth as soon as you notice it appearing so that only *you* need know.

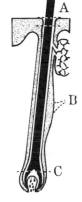

Here is what happens when you remove hair by the various methods:

A. Shave and you remove the hair on the surface of the skin. The blunted end will gradually grow out making the hair appear to be thicker.

B. Depilatory creams remove hair below the surface of the skin.

C. Depilatory wax plucks hair from further down so it takes longer for any remaining hair to reach the skin's surface.

Today's special treatment
Place a looking glass where you can view yourself in clear daylight. Any unwanted hair? Tackle it now. Bleach, shave or use a depilatory cream or wax, then dab on baby cream or a mild all-purpose cream. No unwanted hair? Turn back to Day 3. It's time for another salon facial.

Cleanse, tone, moisturize
Cleanse, tone and moisturize your face in the morning and at night. If you are removing facial hair, make sure skin is clean before you start your treatment and apply a mild cream afterwards.

Elbows
Still rough or discoloured? Mix lemon juice with a little salt and rub in. Rinse off after 5 to 10 minutes and apply body lotion.

Dinginess?
Blend hand cream with 6 drops of 10-volume peroxide and smooth it into dingy areas on thighs or under arms.

Goosepimples?
Lather goosepimply areas with a soft brush. Splash with cold water, pat dry and rub in cream or body lotion.

Hair livener
Massage scalp, see page 61, Day 7, but omit oil.

Shopping Checklist Day 11

Choose your meals, then write in by each relevant item the amount you require.

Amount required	Amount required	Amount required
Fruit and Vegetables	Low-fat fruit yogurt	Wholemeal bread
Cabbage	Low-fat natural yogurt	**Store cupboard**
Courgettes	Low-fat spread	Caraway seeds
Leeks	Skimmed milk	Drinking chocolate
Mushrooms	**Grocery**	Low-calorie salad
Onion	Baked beans in	dressing
Parsley	tomato sauce	Marmalade or jam
Spinach	Bran breakfast cereal	Salt and pepper
Tomatoes	Crispbreads	Sugar
Watercress	Crusty roll	Vinegar
Cooking apple	Flaked almonds	Yeast extract
Grapes	Fruit cocktail in	
Lemon	apple juice or low-	
Orange	calorie syrup	
Strawberries or	Ginger nuts or	
raspberries	malted milk biscuits	
Frozen Food	Lemon juice	
Ice cream	Low-calorie soup	
Spinach	Meringue nest or	
Strawberries or	basket	
raspberries	Parsley & thyme	
Meat, Poultry and Fish	stuffing mix	
Haddock fillets	Pineapple in	
Trout	natural juice	
Dairy Produce/Eggs	Sultanas	
Eggs	Walnuts	

Diet Day 11

☐ 275ml/½ pint skimmed milk or reconstituted low-fat powdered milk

BREAKFAST/SUPPER MEAL

Either ☐ 150g/5.3oz can baked beans in tomato sauce; 1 small slice wholemeal bread, 25g/1oz, toasted

Or ☐ 25g/1oz any bran breakfast cereal; 75ml/5 level tablespoons skimmed milk; 6 grapes

Or ☐ 2 small slices wholemeal bread, 25g/1oz each; 10ml/2 level teaspoons low-fat spread; 10ml/2 level teaspoons marmalade or jam

LIGHT MEAL

Either to eat at home
Egg Florentine plus Fruit

☐ 175g/6oz spinach, fresh or frozen
1 egg, size 3
2 crispbreads
10ml/2 level teaspoons yeast extract

1 medium orange
30ml/2 tablespoons low-fat natural yogurt

Chop and cook fresh spinach; cook frozen spinach as instructed. Drain well. Poach egg in water or in a non-stick poacher without fat. Top spinach with egg and serve with crispbreads, spread with yeast extract. Follow with peeled and sliced orange topped with yogurt.

Or to take to work
Crispbreads and Egg Spread plus Fruit

☐ 1 egg, size 3
Few sprigs watercress
15ml/1 tablespoon low-calorie salad dressing

Salt and pepper
4 crispbreads
1 medium orange

Hard boil egg and chop. Chop watercress and mix with egg, salad dressing and seasoning. Take to work in a container and spread on crispbreads. Follow with orange.

Either a quick recipe **Grilled Trout with Almonds plus Fruit and Meringue**

175g/6oz trout
10ml/2 level teaspoons flaked almonds
2 tomatoes
115g/4oz mushrooms
Lemon wedge

200g/7oz can fruit cocktail in apple juice or low-calorie syrup
1 meringue nest or basket
30ml/2 level tablespoons natural yogurt

Grill trout for about 5 minutes on each side. Toast almonds and grill tomatoes. Poach mushrooms in stock. Sprinkle almonds on trout and serve with lemon wedge, tomatoes and mushrooms. Drain the fruit and top with crushed meringue and yogurt.

Or a keen cook's recipe **Stuffed Haddock plus Strawberry Meringue and Ice Cream**

200g/7oz haddock fillets
45ml/3 level tablespoons parsley and thyme stuffing mix
10ml/2 teaspoons lemon juice
15ml/1 level tablespoon fresh parsley
1 tomato
115g/4oz cabbage

Caraway seeds (optional)
2 small leeks or courgettes
1 meringue nest or basket
50g/2oz strawberries or raspberries, fresh or frozen
1 small scoop vanilla ice cream, 25g/1oz

Put half fish, skin side down, in a small ovenproof dish. Mix stuffing mix and lemon juice with boiling water to form a stiff mixture. Allow to stand for 5 minutes. Stir in parsley and spread mixture on the fish. Top with remaining fish, skin side upwards. Arrange sliced tomato on top. Cover with foil and bake at 180°C/350°F, gas mark 4, for about 40 minutes. Finely slice and boil cabbage adding caraway seeds for seasoning if you wish. Slice and boil the leeks or courgettes. Serve vegetables with fish. Put the meringue nest in a dish and top with strawberries or raspberries and serve with ice cream.

Or if you prefer to eat vegetarian **Sweet and Sour Cabbage plus Yogurt**

115g/4oz cooking apple
75g/3oz onion
175g/6oz red or white cabbage
5ml/1 level teaspoon sugar
Salt and pepper
45ml/3 tablespoons vinegar
30ml/2 tablespoons water
15ml/1 level tablespoon sultanas

50g/2oz canned pineapple in natural juice
15g/½oz walnuts
30ml/2 tablespoons low-fat natural yogurt
1 small low-fat fruit yogurt, any flavour

Peel and chop apple and onion. Finely shred cabbage and put into a saucepan with apple, onion, sugar, vinegar, water and seasoning to taste. Cover and cook over a very low heat for 30 minutes. Stir occasionally and add a little more water if necessary to prevent sticking. Stir in sultanas and chopped pineapple. Cover again and continue to simmer for 10-15 minutes. Stir in chopped walnuts, turn out onto a serving dish and top with natural yogurt. Follow with the fruit yogurt.

Snack 1 ☐ *150ml/¼ pint skimmed milk*   *4 ginger nuts or malted milk*
20ml/2 rounded teaspoons   *biscuits*
    drinking chocolate

Snack 2 ☐ *1 can low-calorie soup, any*   *10ml/2 level teaspoons low-*
    flavour   *fat spread*
1 crusty roll, brown or white

☐ If you completed the day without cheating at all, tick here and move on to Day 12.

☐ If you cheated, do a 'Saintly Day' tomorrow (page 253) instead of the set menu.

☐ If you do not eat one meal or snack that you are allowed, tick this box and save up for a 'Naughty Day'. When you have two ticks saved, you can do any of the Thoroughly Naughty Day's Menus *instead* of your next day's diet.

Exercise Day 11

MORNING ☐ Repeat Exercise 1: 5 times

☐ Repeat Exercise 2: 5 times to right
5 times to left

☐ Repeat Exercise 3: 5 times circling left and right with right foot
5 times circling left and right with left foot

☐ Repeat Exercise 4: touch the floor 15 times

☐ Repeat Exercise 5: bend to the left and right 15 times

☐ Repeat Exercise 6: circle to left 15 times
circle to right 15 times

Exercise 7 ☐ Lie down on the floor with arms parallel with body.
Put feet flat on floor with knees bent. Raise knees to chest
and stretch legs up at right angles to body. Swing legs
wide apart and make scissor movements by crossing one
leg in front of the other. Criss-cross 5 times, then return
slowly to starting position.

LUNCHTIME ☐ Walk for 15 minutes. Turn and return the same way in 12
minutes.

EVENING ☐ Run to the top of the stairs and down again 3 times. Jog for
6 minutes.

Or ☐ Jog for 12 minutes.

Bedtime Relaxer ☐

Beauty Day 11

Don't forget your back view!

Your hair
Check your hair from the back as well as from the front. If
you decide to have it cut shorter or to sweep it up, be sure
that you are not revealing more than you intended: colour
retouching needed at roots, undetected spots at back of
neck, ears which perhaps are better hidden?

Your back

This is one of skin's oilier areas so don't be surprised if you discover some spots. Just get to work to reduce the oiliness with today's special treatment. Itchy back? Skin can react to fibres, such as wool, which may aggravate spots. Overcome this by wearing a soft shirt between you and the scratcher. A tinted body make-up will help to camouflage spots if you're going 'backless' but, unless it's a medicated brand, you should dab on antiseptic before applying.

Your bottom

Dieting can take off unwanted inches and the exercise on page 148, Day 18 helps to tone sagging bottom muscles. Jeans made from stretch fabrics support and shape. Look for those sectioned and seamed from below the belt but try on and view from *all* angles before you buy.

Your legs

We discuss these in more detail on page 219, Day 26, but meanwhile check backs of thighs for hair growth as it is so easily missed. Rub body cream into roughened ankles every night for the next week.

Today's special treatment

Relax shoulders and fend off ageing stiffness. Sit comfortably and *slowly* lift and lower shoulders. Bring them forward as you lift, draw them back as you lower. Do it for a few minutes every day from now on.

Back smoother

Treat an oily, spotty back this way: soak in a warm bath for 5 to 10 minutes and scrub back with a bath brush and medicated soap. Rinse well, pat dry and dab with diluted antiseptic. Then fluff on medicated talc. Do this every night for a week, then on alternate nights until the spots disappear.

Cleanse, tone, moisturize

Cleanse, tone and moisturize your face in the morning and at night.

Hair livener

For dry hair only: massage scalp, see page 61, Day 7, but omit oil.

Roughened ankles?

Massage with body cream.

Blackheads?

Repeat steam treatment from page 42, Day 4.

Shopping Checklist Day 12

Choose your meals, then write in by each relevant item the amount you require.

Amount required		Amount required	
Fruit and Vegetables		**Grocery**	
Broccoli		Bran breakfast cereal	
Celery		Brown rice	
Cucumber		Canned tomatoes	
French beans		Crispbreads	
Lettuce		Crumpets	
Mustard and cress		Low-calorie soup	
Banana		Raisins or sultanas	
Oranges		Sweetcorn	
Pear		Wholemeal bread	
Frozen Foods		**Store cupboard**	
Broccoli		Cornflour	
French beans		Honey	
Sweetcorn		Mixed herbs	
Meat, Poultry and Fish		Oil-free French	
Cooked ham		dressing	
Dairy Produce/Eggs		Salt and pepper	
Butter or margarine		Worcestershire sauce	
Cheese spread			
Cottage cheese			
Edam or Tendale cheese			
Eggs			
Low-fat spread			
Skimmed milk			

Diet Day 12

275ml/½ pint skimmed milk or reconstituted low-fat powdered milk

BREAKFAST/SUPPER MEAL

Either
1 slice wholemeal bread, 40g/1½oz; 1 egg, size 3; 5ml/1 level teaspoon low-fat spread.
Dip bread in beaten egg and fry in a non-stick pan greased with low-fat spread.

Or
25g/1oz any bran breakfast cereal; 75ml/5 tablespoons skimmed milk; 15ml/1 level tablespoon raisins or sultanas

Or
2 small slices wholemeal bread, 25g/1oz each; Half small can tomatoes; Worcestershire sauce; Salt and pepper
Toast bread; heat tomatoes and season with Worcestershire sauce and salt and pepper. Serve tomatoes on toast.

LIGHT MEAL

Either to eat at home
Soup plus Ham and Cheese Salad

1 small can any low-calorie soup	Lettuce
50g/2oz cooked ham	Mustard & cress
50g/2oz cottage cheese with pineapple	2 crispbreads

Heat soup. Remove any visible fat from ham and serve with cottage cheese and a salad of lettuce, and mustard and cress. Eat crispbreads with soup or salad.

Or to take to work
Soup plus Ham and Cheese Sandwich and Pear

1 sachet low-calorie instant soup, any flavour	25g/1oz ham
2 small slices wholemeal bread, 25g/1oz each	1 triangle cheese spread, 15g/½oz
	1 medium pear

Take soup to work in a flask or mix there. Remove all visible fat from ham and make into a sandwich with bread and cheese spread. Follow with pear.

Or if you prefer to eat vegetarian
Caribbean Rice Salad

40g/1½oz brown rice	15ml/1 level tablespoon raisins
2 small oranges	
1 small banana	

Cook rice in boiling water. Rinse in cold water and drain.

Peel and segment one orange and squeeze juice from the second one. Slice banana. Mix rice with fruit and add raisins and orange juice and mix well.

MAIN MEAL

Either a quick recipe **Sweetcorn Omelet and Cheese and Crispbread** ☐

50g/2oz sweetcorn, frozen or canned
2 eggs, size 3
15ml/1 tablespoon skimmed milk
Salt and pepper
Pinch mixed herbs

5ml/1 level teaspoon butter or margarine
150g/5oz French beans or broccoli
25g/1oz Edam or Tendale cheese
1 crispbread

Cook the frozen sweetcorn or heat the canned corn. Beat eggs with milk and seasonings and cook in a non-stick omelet pan greased with butter or margarine, until just set. Top omelet with corn and fold over. Serve with boiled broccoli and beans. Follow with cheese and crispbread.

Or a keen cook's recipe **Sweetcorn Soufflé and Salad** ☐

50g/2oz sweetcorn, frozen or canned
15ml/1 level tablespoon butter or margarine
15ml/1 level tablespoon cornflour
75ml/3fl oz skimmed milk
2 eggs, size 3
Salt and pepper

5ml/1 level teaspoon low-fat spread
Lettuce
Cucumber
Celery
15ml/1 tablespoon oil-free French dressing

Boil sweetcorn. Melt butter in a small pan. Mix milk and cornflour until smooth and pour into the pan. Stirring all the time, bring to the boil. Separate eggs and beat yolks and seasoning into milk. Fold in sweetcorn. Whisk the egg whites until stiff and fold into sweetcorn mixture. Pour into an ovenproof dish, greased with low-fat spread, and bake at 180°C/350°F, gas mark 4, for about 20 minutes until risen and set. Serve soufflé with a salad made of lettuce, cucumber and celery sprinkled with oil-free French dressing.

Snack 1 ☐

113g/4oz carton cottage cheese, any flavour

2 crispbreads

Snack 2 ☐

2 crumpets, toasted
15ml/1 level tablespoon low-fat spread

10ml/2 teaspoons honey

☐ If you completed the day without cheating at all, tick here and move on to Day 13.

☐ If you cheated, do a 'Saintly Day' tomorrow (page 253) instead of the set menu.

☐ If you do not eat one meal or snack that you are allowed, tick this box and save up for a 'Naughty Day'. When you have two ticks saved, you can do any of the Thoroughly Naughty Day's Menus *instead* of your next day's diet.

Exercise Day 12

MORNING ☐ Repeat Exercise 1: 5 times

☐ Repeat Exercise 2: 5 times to right
5 times to left

☐ Repeat Exercise 3: 5 times circling left and right with right foot
5 times circling left and right with left foot

☐ Repeat Exercise 4: touch the floor 15 times

☐ Repeat Exercise 5: bend to the left and right 15 times

☐ Repeat Exercise 6: circle to left 15 times
circle to right 15 times

☐ Repeat Exercise 7: criss-cross 10 times
Come on, spread those legs really wide in a big V-shape. Toes should point outwards following the line and angle of your leg. Knees should not bend, keep legs really straight and stretched.

LUNCHTIME ☐ Walk for 16 minutes. Turn and return the same way in 13 minutes.

EVENING ☐ Run to the top of the stairs and down again 3 times. Jog for 7 minutes.

Or ☐ Jog for 13 minutes.

Bedtime Relaxer ☐

Beauty Day 12

Changing your eyebrows can change your whole facial expression. Nature usually gets the balance basically right so it is not a good idea to alter the shape of your brows too radically. They may need some reshaping, though, so check with the sketch below. Get rid of stragglers, the tiny hairs which grow *below* the brow line and near nose, but resist the temptation to tweeze above brows. There's no truly painless way to pluck, but a face flannel squeezed out in hot water and pressed against brows can help ease the agony. Stretch the skin outwards until it's taut while tweezering. Splash brows with cold water afterwards and stroke on a little mild medicated cream.

Tweezers come in all shapes and sizes with tips which are narrow, broad, flat and pointed. They're often sold tightly sealed, which makes it impossible to try before you buy, but those with a flat, thin blunted tip are probably the easiest to handle.

Today's special treatment
Shaping your eyebrows (see sketch):

1. Inner brow should begin immediately above inner eye.

2. Look straight ahead. The highest point of your brow should be sited at outer edge of your iris.

3. Measure for the point where brow should end with a slim, long-handled brush or pencil, as in sketch.

Cleanse, tone, moisturize
Cleanse, tone and moisturize your face in the morning and at night.

Hair livener
Massage scalp, see page 61, Day 7, but omit oil.

Roughened ankles?
Massage with body cream.

Spotty back?
Soak in warm bath; scrub back with medicated soap, dry and dab with diluted antiseptic. Dust with medicated talc.

Shopping Checklist Day 13

Choose your meals, then write in by each relevant item the amount you require.

Amount required	*Amount required*	*Amount required*
Fruit and Vegetables	**Dairy Produce/Eggs**	Low-calorie
Cabbage	Cottage cheese with	seafood sauce
Carrots	pineapple	Stock cube
Celery	Curd cheese	
Lettuce	Egg	
Onion	Grated parmesan	
Peas	cheese	
Potatoes	Low-fat natural	
Spinach	yogurt	
Tomatoes	Low-fat spread	
Banana	Skimmed milk	
Orange	**Grocery**	
Peach	Bran breakfast cereal	
Frozen Foods	Crispbreads	
Cod steak in	Digestive biscuit	
parsley sauce	Dried stoned dates	
Mixed vegetables	Peach canned in	
Peas	natural juice,	
Spinach	low-calorie syrup	
Meat, Poultry and Fish	or water	
Lamb chop	Unsweetened orange	
Pork chop	juice	
Prawns	Wholemeal bread	
Streaky bacon	**Store cupboard**	
	Cinnamon	
	Honey	

Diet Day 13

☐ *275ml/½ pint skimmed milk or reconstituted low-fat powdered milk*

BREAKFAST/SUPPER

Either ☐ *2 tomatoes, grilled without fat; 2 rashers streaky bacon, well grilled; 1 small slice wholemeal bread, 25g/1oz*

Or ☐ *1 egg, size 3, boiled; 1 small slice wholemeal bread, 25g/1oz; 5ml/1 level teaspoon low-fat spread*

Or ☐ *25g/1oz any bran breakfast cereal; 75ml/5 tablespoons skimmed milk; 1 small orange*

LIGHT MEAL

Either to eat at home **Cod in Parsley Sauce** ☐ *1 frozen cod steak in parsley sauce   115g/4oz peas, frozen   2 tomatoes*
Cook the cod in sauce as directed. Boil the peas and grill tomatoes without fat. Serve vegetables with cod.

Or to take to work **Prawn Sandwich plus Orange** ☐ *2 small slices wholemeal bread, 25g/1oz each   15ml/1 tablespoon low-calorie seafood sauce*
Lettuce   Salt and pepper
50g/2oz shelled prawns   1 small orange
Shred lettuce and put between the bread slices. Mix prawns, dressing and seasoning in a small container and take to work separately. At work, make up the sandwich. Follow with the orange.

Or if you prefer to eat vegetarian **Fruity Cottage Cheese Crispbreads** ☐ *1 small banana   2 crispbreads*
113g/4oz carton cottage cheese with pineapple
Slice banana and mix with cottage cheese. Eat with crispbreads.

*Either a
quick recipe*
**Grilled Lamb
Chop plus
Peach Dessert**

175g/6oz lamb chop
75g/3oz mixed vegetables,
    frozen
115g/4oz potato
6 peach slices, fresh or
    canned in natural juice,
    low-calorie syrup or water

1 small digestive biscuit
45ml/3 level tablespoons low-
    fat natural yogurt

Remove all visible fat from chop and grill. Boil mixed
vegetables and potato. Serve chop topped with 3 drained
peach slices and vegetables. To follow: put the remaining
peach slices in a small dish. Crumble biscuit, mix with yogurt
and use to top peach slices.

---

*Or a keen
cook's recipe*
**Braised Pork
Chop plus
Spicy Baked
Peach**

175g/6oz pork chop
115g/4oz red or white
    cabbage
1 small onion
150ml/¼ pint stock made
    with ½ stock cube
1 peach, fresh or canned in
    natural juice, low-calorie
    syrup or water

Salt and pepper
115g/4oz potato
Cinnamon
30ml/2 tablespoons peach
    juice or unsweetened
    orange juice

Remove all visible fat from chop and grill for a few minutes
on each side. Thinly slice cabbage and onion and layer in a
small ovenproof dish. Put chop on top of vegetables and
pour over stock. Chop half the peach and add to the dish.
Season. Cover with lid or foil and bake at 180°C/350°F, gas
mark 4, for about 45 minutes until the meat is tender. Serve
with boiled potato. Put second half of peach in an ovenproof
dish and sprinkle with cinnamon. Spoon over fruit juice and
bake at 180°C/350°F, gas mark 4, for 15 minutes.

---

*Or if you
prefer to eat
vegetarian*
**Spinach and
Carrot Bake
plus Banana
and Dates**

175g/6oz spinach, fresh or
    frozen
115g/4oz carrots
1 egg, size 3
150ml/¼ pint skimmed milk

30ml/2 level tablespoons
    grated Parmesan cheese
Salt and pepper
1 medium banana
25g/1oz dried stoned dates

Cook fresh spinach until tender; drain and chop. Defrost
frozen spinach and drain. Grate carrot. Beat egg into the
milk, add cheese and season. Mix egg mixture with carrot
and spinach and put into an ovenproof dish. Bake at
160°C/325°F, gas mark 3, for 45 minutes or until set and the
top is brown. Follow with sliced banana mixed with chopped
dates.

Snack 1 ☐   2 small slices wholemeal   10ml/2 level teaspoons low-
                    bread, 25g/1oz each,   fat spread
                    toasted   20ml/4 level teaspoons honey

Snack 2 ☐   115g/4oz curd cheese   2 crispbreads
                    4 sticks celery

☐ If you completed the day without cheating at all, tick here and move on to Day 14.

☐ If you cheated, do a 'Saintly Day' tomorrow (page 253) instead of the set menu.

☐ If you do not eat one meal or snack that you are allowed, tick this box and save up for a 'Naughty Day'.
When you have two ticks saved, you can do any of the Thoroughly Naughty Day's Menus *instead* of your next day's diet.

Exercise Day 13

MORNING ☐ Repeat Exercise 1: 5 times

☐ Repeat Exercise 2: 5 times to right
5 times to left

☐ Repeat Exercise 3: 5 times circling left and right with right foot
5 times circling left and right with left foot

☐ Repeat Exercise 4: touch the floor 15 times

☐ Repeat Exercise 5: bend to the left and right 15 times

☐ Repeat Exercise 6: circle to left 15 times
circle to right 15 times

☐ Repeat Exercise 7: criss-cross 15 times

As the exercise session now takes more of your time, you may like to choose some of the exercises to do at lunchtime and some in the evening. It doesn't matter when you do the exercises but don't put them off until tomorrow. It is important to get into the daily exercise habit.

LUNCHTIME ☐ Walk for 17 minutes. Turn and return the same way in 14 minutes.

EVENING ☐ Run to the top of the stairs and down again 4 times. Jog for 7 minutes.

Or ☐ Jog for 14 minutes.

Bedtime Relaxer ☐

Beauty Day 13

Hairstyle, make-up and well-cut uncluttered clothes can help a woman to look young and attractive. Here are a few other ways to keep the years at bay.

Treasure your skin
The fibres which support it may lose some of their resilience as the years go by. You can't stop that but you can fight back with regular skin care and extra treats for the parts which are usually the first to show signs of wear and tear.

Around the eyes
The muscles which control eye movements make ageing demands on this area, so it makes sense to cream often to help delay lines. Eye creams are especially light but are usually expensive, and moisturizer can be used instead. Fingerprint cream in very lightly taking care not to stretch the skin around the eyes.

For droopy lids the make-up on page 166, Day 20, plays clever tricks.

Around the mouth
You may see downward nose to mouth lines here. Massage with moisturizer regularly and repeat the home facial we featured on page 37, Day 3.

On the neck
Your neck is a give-away when it begins to look 'crepey'.
It's short on natural oil glands to keep it supple, so give it a
twice-weekly treat (see page 49, Day 5). Disguise a neck
problem by wearing a high, soft frilly neckline. It's
softening for the face, too.

Today's special treatment
Exercises to tone facial muscles.

Cheeky ☐ Puff out cheeks and blow as hard as you can without letting
any air escape from between your lips. Breathe naturally
through your nose. You should feel the pressure inside your
cheeks. Hold for a slow count of 3. Relax. Puff 2 or 3 times
more.

Nestling ☐ Open your mouth and allow your head to drop backwards,
rather like a baby bird. Close your mouth and feel the
tension below your chin. Open and close your mouth 3 more
times, slowly. Bring back your head to its normal position.

Are you a ☐ Remember to walk and sit gracefully (page 74, Day 8).
young mover?

Cleanse, tone, ☐ Cleanse, tone and moisturize your face in the morning and
moisturize at night.

Elbows ☐ Still rough or discoloured? Mix lemon juice with a little salt
and rub in. Rinse off after 5 to 10 minutes and apply body
lotion.

Dinginess? ☐ Blend hand cream with 6 drops of 10-volume peroxide and
smooth it into dingy areas on thighs or under arms.

Roughened ☐ Massage with body cream.
ankles?

Hair livener ☐ For dry hair only: massage scalp, see page 61, Day 7, but
omit oil.

Spotty back? ☐ Soak in warm bath; scrub back with medicated soap, dry
and dab with diluted antiseptic. Dust with medicated talc.

Shopping Checklist Day 14

Choose your meals, then write in by each relevant item the amount you require.

Amount required	*Amount required*
Fruit and Vegetables	**Grocery**
Brussels sprouts	Bran breakfast cereal
Carrot	Cheese sauce mix
Lettuce	Crispbreads
Mushrooms	Currant bun
Onion	Dried apricot halves
Potato	Low-fat skimmed
Tomatoes	milk powder
Apple	Low-calorie tartare
Banana	sauce or salad
Pear	dressing
Frozen Foods	Pasta shells
Brussels sprouts	Sweetcorn
Sweetcorn	Wholemeal bread
Meat, Poultry and Fish	**Store cupboard**
Chicken or turkey	Cornflour
Corned beef	Marmalade or jam
Dairy Produce/Eggs	Salt and pepper
Edam or Tendale	Stock cube
cheese	Sweet pickle
Eggs	Yeast extract
Low-fat natural	
yogurt	
Low-fat spread	
Skimmed milk	

Diet Day 14

☐ 275ml/½ pint skimmed milk or reconstituted low-fat powdered milk

BREAKFAST/SUPPER MEAL

Either ☐ *2 eggs, size 3; 15ml/1 tablespoon skimmed milk; 1 tomato*
Scramble eggs with milk and serve with tomato grilled without fat.

Or ☐ *25g/1oz any bran breakfast cereal; 60ml/4 tablespoons low-fat natural yogurt; 2 dried apricot halves, chopped*

Or ☐ *2 small slices wholemeal bread, 25g/1oz each, toasted; 10ml/2 level teaspoons low-fat spread; 10ml/2 level teaspoons marmalade or jam*

LIGHT MEAL

Either to eat at home
Corned Beef and Mashed Potato
☐ *115g/4oz potato*   *50g/2oz corned beef*
15ml/1 tablespoon skimmed milk   *15ml/1 level tablespoon sweet pickle*
Salt and pepper
Boil potato and mash it with milk and seasoning. Serve with corned beef and pickle.

Or to take to work
Corned Beef and Pickle Sandwich
☐ *2 small slices wholemeal bread, 25g/1oz each*   *25ml/1 tablespoon sweet pickle*
50g/2oz corned beef   *2 tomatoes*
Make sandwich with bread, corned beef and pickle. Take tomatoes separately to eat with sandwich.

Or if you prefer to eat vegetarian
Stuffed Tomatoes and Crispbread
☐ *2 tomatoes*   *Salt and pepper*
1 egg, size 3   *Lettuce*
15ml/1 level tablespoon low-calorie tartare sauce or salad dressing   *3 crispbreads*
15ml/1 level tablespoon low-fat spread
Cut top off each tomato and carefully scoop out pulp. Save pulp to add to the next soup or casserole you make. Stand tomato shell upside down to drain. Hard-boil the egg and chop. Mix with tartare sauce or salad dressing and season to

taste. Spoon egg mixture into tomato shells and serve with shredded lettuce and crispbreads scraped with low-fat spread.

MAIN MEAL

Either a quick recipe
Roast Chicken or Turkey Dinner plus Apple

75g/3oz roast chicken or turkey, skin removed
150g/5oz roast potatoes, large chunks
115g/4oz Brussels sprouts, boiled

115g/4oz carrots, boiled
30ml/2 tablespoons fatless gravy
1 medium apple

Or a keen cook's recipe
Chicken or Turkey Breast with Mushroom Sauce plus Banana

150g/5oz raw boned chicken or turkey breast, skin removed
150ml/¼ pint stock made from ½ chicken stock cube
25g/1oz onion
50g/2oz mushrooms
5ml/1 level teaspoon low-fat spread

10ml/2 level teaspoons cornflour
30ml/2 level tablespoons dried low-fat milk powder
Salt and pepper
115g/4oz Brussels sprouts
115g/4oz carrots
1 medium banana

Place chicken or turkey breast in a small saucepan with stock, onion and mushrooms. Bring to the boil, cover and simmer gently for 30 minutes. Remove meat and mushrooms and keep warm. Drain liquid into a measuring jug and make up to 150ml/5floz with water. Pour into a saucepan and add the low-fat spread, cornflour and milk powder. Bring to the boil, whisking all the time and cook for 2-3 minutes. Season to taste and stir in the mushrooms. Pour sauce over the breast and serve with boiled vegetables. Follow with banana.

Or if you prefer to eat vegetarian
Cheesy Pasta and Sweetcorn plus Pear

115g/4oz sweetcorn, canned or frozen
25g/1oz pasta shells
½ packet cheese sauce mix
150ml/¼ pint skimmed milk

1 tomato
Salt and pepper
25g/1oz Edam or Tendale cheese
1 pear

Cook frozen sweetcorn or drain canned. Cook pasta in boiling salted water until just tender. Make cheese sauce using skimmed milk. Slice tomato, reserve three slices and chop remainder. Add cooked sweetcorn, pasta and chopped tomato to cheese sauce. Warm through, season and turn into a small ovenproof dish. Grate cheese and sprinkle on dish and top with reserved tomato slices. Grill for a few minutes until cheese browns. Follow with pear.

Snack 1 ☐
2 crispbreads
10ml/2 teaspoons yeast
    extract

40g/1½oz Edam or Tendale
    cheese
2 tomatoes

Spread crispbreads with yeast extract. Top with cheese and tomatoes.

Snack 2 ☐
1 currant bun
10ml/2 level teaspoons low-
    fat spread

1 small banana

☐ If you completed the day without cheating at all, tick here and move on to Day 15.

☐ If you cheated, do a 'Saintly Day' tomorrow (page 253) instead of the set menu.

☐ If you do not eat one meal or snack that you are allowed, tick this box and save up for a 'Naughty Day'.
When you have two ticks saved, you can do any of the Thoroughly Naughty Day's Menus *instead* of your next day's diet.

Exercise Day 14

MORNING ☐ Repeat Exercise 1: 5 times

☐ Repeat Exercise 2: 5 times to right
5 times to left

☐ Repeat Exercise 3: 5 times circling left and right with right foot
5 times circling left and right with left foot

☐ Repeat Exercise 4: touch the floor 15 times

☐ Repeat Exercise 5: bend to the left and right 15 times

☐ Repeat Exercise 6: circle to left 15 times
circle to right 15 times

☐ Repeat Exercise 7: criss-cross 20 times.
Relax for a few moments before continuing with the next exercise.

Exercise 8 ☐ Lie on floor with body in a straight line and arms by sides. Keeping arms straight, swing them up and over head to touch the floor behind. Feel the spine stretching. Repeat 4 more times.

LUNCHTIME ☐ Walk for 18 minutes. Turn and return the same way in 15 minutes.

EVENING ☐ Run to the top of the stairs and down again 4 times. Jog for 8 minutes.

Or ☐ Jog for 15 minutes.

If you cannot manage this amount of jogging all at once, break it into 5-minute jogs to do whenever you wish and tick them below!

1st 5-minute jog
2nd 5-minute jog
3rd 5-minute jog

Bedtime Relaxer ☐

Beauty Day 14

Now it's time to take a fresh look at yourself: if you have been following our beauty plan your skin should be smoother, clearer, less oily or less dry.

Did you try the oily skin treatments?
Carry on with the soap and water lathering, page 42, Day 4. It will help control oiliness and reduce the risk of

blackheads. If you have no noticeable blackheads or spots, steam your face once a week only from now on. Any taut, dry patches? Ask your chemist for a soothing medicated cream. If the patches persist, your skin may be drier in some areas than you thought and you should avoid those parts when de-oiling.

Did you try the dry skin treatment?
Your skin should feel softer, but if your oil glands are low producers you will probably need to continue compensating for them. On the coldest, driest days try this before you put on your make-up: smooth in moisturizer, leave for 10 minutes, then smooth in some more. Wait another 10 minutes before applying foundation. Do you sometimes squeeze out a little too much hand cream? Don't waste it! Stroke lightly upward over your neck; or cup palms and rub over elbows.

Hands dry and dingy?
The drier they are, the dingier they seem, but washing makes them drier — it's a vicious circle. So if your hands have been slow to respond to care, mix up some pastry — but not for eating! Mix 1oz to 2oz of fat with a generous pinch of salt and a heaped tablespoon of flour. Rub well into hands for 10 minutes before throwing it away. Rinse hands and you will probably be surprised at how much cleaner and softer they are.

Today's special treatment
Repeat the all-over 'spring clean' (page 22, Day 1) then tone skin once more with a face mask; use one from page 43, Day 4 or *Cupboard Love* below. Relax as you would in a luxurious salon. Slip into something flimsy, warm and comfortable. Put your feet up and lie back.

Cupboard Love Beauty Mask

Mix a teaspoon each of clear honey and plain yogurt with an egg yolk. Blend with a little powdered milk if it's very runny. Smooth mask over face and leave on for 10-15 minutes before rinsing off with warm, then cool water. It's a gentle mix so it should suit most skin types.

Cleanse, tone, moisturize

Cleanse, tone and moisturize before applying make-up. If your skin is dry, apply moisturizer after your beauty mask treatment.

Roughened ankles?

Rub body cream into ankles after 'spring clean' treatment.

Hair livener   ☐   Massage scalp, see page 61, Day 7, but omit oil.

Reassess your skin   ☐   Make sure that you are following the correct treatments for your skin. Tomorrow morning, before you wash, press a large tissue firmly over your face. Then examine it for oiliness.

☐   If there are extensive oily patches, you can assume you have an oily skin, so tick this box.

☐   An oily strip only in the centre area suggests that you have combined oily and dry skin.

☐   A trace of oil at the centre shows that your skin is normal.

☐   If the tissue is oil-free, your skin is dry.

How to make your own luck

'Lucky old Beverley. Good things always seem to happen to her. She's one of those naturally lucky people.' We bet you've heard that sentiment expressed countless times.

Now it's very important to get this thing called 'luck' into proper perspective. We all know seemingly 'lucky' people. The type who appear to have a direct line to a smiling fate, who possess the knack of turning every tiny happy event to immense personal advantage, who determinedly place themselves in positions of strength where they can realize their human potential easily and confidently . . . The people who, in short, live their lives blissfully to the full. So when you meet one of these 'lucky' people and feel immediately dazzled by her self-confidence and success, it's fairly natural to feel that life has short-changed you. Particularly if you're going through a gruelling patch. You may have marital problems, job difficulties, financial worries or just feel generally low. If this is the case, it's very easy to indulge in the fantasy that fate delights in taking huge swipes at you, at the same time benevolently distributing the choicest pickings of life to others.

This concept of luck is total fantasy. To a great extent each of us is responsible for our own luck in life. Dig deep enough within the stereotyped 'lucky' person and you'll find talent in the widest sense of the word — plus, perhaps more importantly, an impressive track record of sheer perseverance and the courage to go one's own way. Because those people who appear to have won what they want out of life have had, at some stage, to make the same decisions which possibly face you. We're talking about (1) defining what you want from life, (2) taking your courage in both hands, and (3) making the best attempt you can to achieve what you desire.

Sounds easy, doesn't it? In fact, deciding exactly what you want and then working on a set of goals in order to achieve it, is often one of the hardest tasks which face us. For a start, you need to be ruthless with yourself. You have to examine what you can give to the world and decide honestly what you can hope to expect from it. This is because, to some extent, the mechanics of luck are like money: get the basic investments right and it will begin to accumulate on its own account. Your plan might then demand re-examination of all your values, attitudes and ideas. Finally, it requires hard work and self-discipline — as many 'lucky' people are quick to point out — to get where you want to go! All things considered, it's often much easier to sit back and moan that all life does is kick you in the teeth, rather than to sit up straight, take stock and deliberately invite changes — with all their attendant risks — into your life.

But let's assume that you want to change your luck — or, more precisely, to put yourself into a position where good things start happening to you. How do you go about it? Being lucky or getting what we want starts with our thoughts and actions: thoughts inspire actions; actions make things happen. This may sound ridiculously elementary, but many intelligent people overlook the fact that it's 'doing' in life — not just 'thinking' about it — that counts. There is a kind of thinking which children tend to indulge in — let's call it 'magical' thinking — which consists of the fantasy that just because one thinks or hopes something will happen, it will magically occur without any direct effort on the individual's part. (You would be surprised how many adults retain this 'magical' thinking all their lives.) So the first step is to discard all 'magical' thoughts, replacing them with thoughts which are likely to inspire positive action. You see, very often the person who experiences a continuous round of bad luck gets bogged down in a range of negative thoughts, which lead to negative behaviour which leads to more bad luck and more negative thinking . . . And the vicious circle is complete. This is the result of a negative self-fulfilling prophecy. A particularly good example of this is the overweight woman who feels so desperately unattractive that she cannot find the energy to make herself even the tiniest bit attractive. She grooms herself poorly, dresses carelessly, avoids contact with the opposite sex and is even ambivalent to her own sex, so nobody is aware she is lonely and willing to be friends. Eventually, she withdraws from the world, justifying her position with irrational, self-pitying thoughts: 'Look how ugly and unattractive I am — no wonder nobody wants me. Nobody cares. And why should they? I really am so unattractive.'

Similarly, a woman may not have a noticeable weight problem but she can still possess a bad or damaged self-image which makes her go around blaming herself continually for all her problems. This is the woman who will mentally talk herself down to the point where any sort of positive action would totally paralyse her. Her daily litany goes something like this: 'I'm just an awful mess. That's why awful things keep happening to me. I know that I will never have any fun or find any satisfaction. But there's nothing I can do to help myself.'

Conversely, there is the woman who blames all her troubles on the rest of the world. She totally denies responsibility for herself and anything that happens to her. Having dumped the responsibility for her own destiny on to the world so completely, when things go wrong or people don't come up to her expectations she backs off with a self-pitying moan: 'I hate this rotten, beastly, unfair world. It's lousy and a horrible place to be. I hate everything in it.' In most cases, this type of woman has an extremely robust self-image but, unfortunately, it works against her — because it blurs true reality and thus prevents the sort of constructive self-examination which could help produce a more balanced mental attitude.

All this illustrates how thoughts and actions relate so intensely, and how our minds, if exposed to a continual battery of negative thoughts, will keep our bodies fettered to a negative environment. It is therefore vitally important to think positively if you want luck to enter your life.

It is pointless moaning that life doesn't present opportunity or excitement if you wrap yourself in cotton wool and never dare to meet its challenges. We're all guilty of this to some extent. But probably the classic illustration is the overweight woman who overeats out of loneliness, then refuses social invitations when they are offered because she feels fat and unattractive. So she stays in night after night, watching TV and eating for comfort.

Having assertive skills simply means being able to make the right requests to the appropriate people, and to make and accept refusals. Each of us has the right to ask anybody to do anything for us. On the other hand, people have the right to refuse us. We have to learn to ask, to make demands of others, to reciprocate when we wish and also, when we feel we must, to refuse the demands made on us. Work on the premise that, to make your own luck in life, you have to learn to ask the world to make room for you.

So the next step is getting accustomed to verbalizing requests: putting your needs into words. Now this is not as simple as it may sound. Very many people find it extremely difficult to make requests, and they imagine — in the same way that children think 'magically' — that, just because the request has formed in their heads, others will be able to mind-read and grant the request automatically. Well, of course, few people possess these kinds of telepathic powers! If you want something from someone, you have to *ask*. Most people are inhibited about making requests because they think that, if they are refused, the person doing the refusing is really saying: 'No, I won't do this for you or you can't have such-an-such a thing because I don't like you as an individual.' Or, worse, that the refusal implies: 'You can't have this request granted because you are not worthy enough.' Yet, 9 times out of 10, no slight or personal affront is intended. If a request is refused, it's for extremely sound, logical reasons. Only our insecurities about our own personalities make us invest a simple refusal with a deep rebuff where none is intended.

To achieve success in life, we have to accept that not everyone is going to approve of who we are or what we want — just as it is unrealistic to expect to win the world's approval all the time or even expect to be liked all the time. We have to learn to accept graciously each 'no' when it comes, as some invariably will, but at the same time refuse to be put off course. And to keep on persisting until we eventually find the 'yes' we seek — for this will assuredly come, too. As 'lucky' people point out, it's persistence that opens doors in life and gets requests granted.

In much the same way that we must learn to develop an attitude to dealing with a 'no', we need to learn something about this other word, 'yes'. You see, there are many ways in which we can say yes to people. There is the whole-hearted yes, with no conditions attached — and there is the qualified yes. It's important to understand the distinction. Here is an example of the unqualified yes. You meet a neighbour on the way home from work who asks if she can borrow the evening newspaper. You say, 'Certainly — go ahead,' and hand over the paper. You wait for the neighbour to return the newspaper as there is something you particularly want to keep in that edition but it isn't forthcoming. Then you get angry and take your annoyance out on anyone else who asks you for anything. 'No' from then on becomes the order of the day. But what you should have told your neighbour was 'Certainly, go ahead. But may I please have it back tomorrow as there's an important item I want to keep.' The neighbour would then have known exactly what was in your mind. This is the proper way to deal with people, being assertive in the real sense of the word.

But there is little point in acquiring the skills of assertion if you don't have a course of action to which you can apply them — and this is where 'goals' come in. We all need goals to structure our expectations and give ourselves a yardstick for achievement. And achievement is vitally important when it comes to making your own luck. We're not talking now about particularly high standards of achievement, just the feeling of satisfaction in accomplishing something we set out to do — however small and seemingly insignificant it may seem to the rest of the world. To feel that you have 'achieved' is a good feeling and one you should allow yourself to experience.

Many people shy away from having goals in life because they tend to set unrealistic or impossibly high standards, then get disappointed when they fail to meet them. The classic example is the grossly overweight person who decides on a goal of losing 4st, then becomes immediately discouraged when the first week's dieting produces only a 2lb loss. Instinctively, the person finds herself saying: 'Only 2lb off — that's 3st 12lb still to go. It's awful. I'll never do it. It's just not worth the effort.' And the diet is abandoned. But if this slimmer had set herself a goal of, say, 2lb a week weight loss, imagine how successful she could feel about that first week: 'I've done it! I've got my calories under control. Now I will set about achieving the same weight loss at the end of next week.' At once, her task seems small, measurable and easily within her power.

If you want to adopt new behaviour patterns, to elicit different responses, you have to be willing to change. This, as it happens, is one of the hardest things to do in life. First, you must want to change enough to take a few risks — because, of course, change always has risks attached to it. There's the chance that the pay-off won't be a positive one and that you might be the loser. Then there is also the realization that, in order to change, you have to leave something of yourself behind — you are in a real sense moving into an unknown future.

You might want to change your life but feel uncertain what to do and which direction to follow. Try to alter the area in your life that is causing you the most unhappiness: whether it's a problem with a spouse, your job, finances, or, of course, your weight. Work positively on that prime problem first and you'll probably find that the changes you put in motion to solve it — whether inside yourself or in your environment — will pay dividends in other areas, too.

Don't be disappointed if it takes some time for your luck to change. There's no cast-iron-guarantee that what we do today will affect events tomorrow or next week — but it might well help to shape the quality of our lives 2, 5 or even 10 years hence.

It's a good feeling to know you have created the luck in your life. So, be assertive, set yourself appropriate goals and be very determined to make your expectations come true. And the very best of luck to you!

Week 3

☐☐ Weigh yourself and write in your weight here

☐☐ Now check the chart on page 7 and write in your ideal weight here

☐☐ Write in the amount you have to lose here

Now tick one of these boxes, and this is your menu plan for this week

☐ If you have under 1st to lose, you can have breakfast/supper, a light meal and a main meal each day.

☐ If you have between 1st and 3st to lose, you can have breakfast/supper, a light meal, a main meal and one snack.

☐ If you have over 3st to lose, you can have breakfast/supper, a light meal, a main meal and two snacks.

Shopping Checklist Day 15

Choose your meals, then write in by each relevant item the amount you require.

Amount required	*Amount required*	*Amount required*
Fruit and Vegetables	**Dairy Produce/Eggs**	Wholemeal bread
Brussels sprouts	Cottage cheese	**Store Cupboard**
Cabbage	Eggs	Black olives
Carrot	Low-fat natural	Cinnamon
Celery	yogurt	Cloves
Garlic	Low-fat spread	Cornflour
Green pepper	Riccotta or curd	Dry cider
Onion	cheese	Ground rice
Potato	Skimmed milk	Low-calorie salad
Spring onions	**Grocery**	dressing
Swede	Apple juice	Liqueur
Tomatoes	Baked beans in	Mixed herbs
Apple	tomato sauce	Oil-free French
Melon	Bran breakfast cereal	dressing
Orange	Broad beans	Salt and pepper
Frozen Foods	Butter beans	Sugar
Broad beans	Chocolate bar	
Brussels sprouts	Crispbreads	
Runner beans	French bread	
Swede	Peanuts	
Sweetcorn	Raisins or sultanas	
Meat, Poultry and Fish	Sardines in tomato	
Chipolata sausages	sauce	
Gammon rasher or	Sweetcorn	
steak	Unsweetened orange	
Ham steak	or pineapple juice	

Diet Day 15

☐ *275ml/½ pint skimmed milk or reconstituted low-fat powdered milk*

BREAKFAST/SUPPER

Either ☐ *1 slice wholemeal bread, 40g/1½oz; 1 egg, size 3; 5ml/1 level teaspoon low-fat spread*
Dip bread into beaten egg and fry in non-stick pan greased with low-fat spread.

Or ☐ *25g/1oz any bran breakfast cereal; 75ml/5 tablespoons skimmed milk; 15ml/1 level tablespoon raisins or sultanas*

Or ☐ *2 beef chipolata sausages, well grilled; 2 tomatoes, grilled without fat; 1 small slice wholemeal bread, 25g/1oz*

LIGHT MEAL

Either to eat at home
Vegetable Hash with Baked Beans

☐ *115g/4oz potato*
115g/4oz swede, fresh or frozen
50g/2oz Brussels sprouts, fresh or frozen

5ml/1 level teaspoon low-fat spread
150g/5.3oz can baked beans in tomato sauce

Boil vegetables then mash and mix together. Season well. Brush a non-stick pan with low-fat spread, then brown hash on each side. Heat beans and serve with vegetable hash.

Or to take to work
Sardine, Apple and Celery Salad

☐ *2 sticks celery*
1 small apple
30ml/2 tablespoons low-calorie salad dressing

2 sardines canned in tomato sauce
2 crispbreads
10ml/2 level teaspoons low-fat spread

Slice celery and dice apple, removing core but leaving skin on. Mix with low-calorie salad dressing and top with sardines. Scrape crispbreads with low-fat spread and take to work separately.

Or if you prefer to eat vegetarian
Mediterranean Bean Salad plus Apple

☐ *213g/7½oz can butter beans*
1 tomato and 1 spring onion
½ green pepper
½ clove garlic

30ml/2 level tablespoons oil-free French dressing
4 black olives, optional
1 medium apple

121

Drain butter beans. Chop tomato, spring onion and pepper. Crush garlic and add to dressing. Toss beans and vegetables in the dressing and garnish with olives. Follow with apple.

MAIN MEAL

Either a quick recipe **Grilled Gammon and Vegetables plus Orange Yogurt**

75g/3oz lean gammon rasher or steak
1 medium orange
115g/4oz broad beans, frozen or canned
75g/3oz sweetcorn, frozen or canned
1 small carton low-fat natural yogurt

Grill gammon rasher or steak. Cut a thin slice from centre of the orange and grill with gammon for last few minutes to warm through. Boil or heat vegetables and serve with gammon and orange. Follow with remaining orange mixed with yogurt.

Or a keen cook's recipe **Ham with Raisin Sauce plus Minty Melon**

99g/3½oz ham steak
5ml/1 level teaspoon brown sugar
1.5ml/½ level teaspoon cornflour
15ml/1 level tablespoon raisins
Pinch cinnamon
2 cloves
75ml/3floz dry cider or apple juice
115g/4oz broad beans, frozen or canned
115g/4oz runner beans
225g/8oz melon
15ml/1 tablespoon crème de menthe or other liqueur

Grill ham steak. To make sauce put sugar, cornflour, raisins, spices and cider or apple juice in saucepan and bring to the boil, stirring all the time. Simmer for 10 minutes. Boil the beans. Remove cloves from sauce and pour it over ham steak. Serve with vegetables. Cut melon into chunks or scoop into balls. Put in a dish and pour over the crème de menthe or any other favourite liqueur. Leave in the refrigerator for at least 30 minutes and serve chilled.

Or if you prefer to eat vegetarian **French Bread Pizza with Coleslaw and Fruity Rice**

50g/2oz French bread
50g/2oz Riccotta or curd cheese
2 tomatoes
Mixed herbs
115g/4oz cabbage
50g/2oz carrot
2 spring onions or ½ small onion
15ml/1 tablespoon low-calorie salad dressing
15ml/1 level tablespoon ground rice
115ml/4fl oz unsweetened orange or pineapple juice
5ml/1 level teaspoon sugar

Cut French bread in half and spread cut surfaces with

cheese. Top with tomato slices and sprinkle with mixed herbs. Grill until cheese starts to melt. Shred cabbage, grate carrot and chop onion. Mix with salad dressing and serve with French bread pizza. Put ground rice and fruit juice into a small saucepan with sugar. Bring to boil, then simmer gently for 2 minutes, stirring all the time, until thick. Serve hot.

Snack 1 ☐ *113g/4oz carton cottage   2 sticks celery cheese, any flavour except 15ml/1 level tablespoon with Cheddar cheese   peanuts*

Snack 2 ☐ *50g/2oz bar chocolate, any brand*

☐ If you completed the day without cheating at all, tick here and move on to Day 16.

☐ If you cheated, do a 'Saintly Day' tomorrow (page 253) instead of the set menu.

☐ If you do not eat one meal or snack that you are allowed, tick this box and save up for a 'Naughty Day'. When you have two ticks saved, you can do any of the Thoroughly Naughty Day's Menus *instead* of your next day's diet.

Exercise Day 15

MORNING ☐ Repeat Exercise 1: 5 times

☐ Repeat Exercise 2: 5 times to right
5 times to left

☐ Repeat Exercise 3: 5 times circling left and right with right foot
5 times circling left and right with left foot

☐ Repeat Exercise 4: touch the floor 15 times

Repeat Exercise 5: bend to the left and right 15 times

Repeat Exercise 6: circle to left 15 times
circle to right 15 times

Repeat Exercise 7: criss-cross 20 times

Repeat Exercise 8: stretch 5 times

Exercise 9   Remain on floor and sit up with legs straight and feet about 3ft apart. Reach up, arms straight above head and bend to touch left ankle or as far down the left leg as you can manage. Hold leg or ankle and gently pull body forward. Return to original position with arms stretched above head and bend to touch right ankle. Repeat 4 more times.

LUNCHTIME   Walk for 19 minutes. Turn and return the same way in 16 minutes.

EVENING   Run to the top of the stairs and down again 4 times. Jog for 9 minutes.

Or   Jog for 16 minutes:
1st 5-minute jog
2nd 5-minute jog
3rd 5-minute jog
4th 1-minute jog

Bedtime Relaxer

Beauty Shopping List Week 3

The number of items you will require depends on your skin type and problems. Check through the week's treatments and write down the products you need to purchase.

Antiseptic	Eyeshadow	Moisturizer
Baby oil	Face powder	Nail clippers or
Blusher	Foundation	scissors
Body lotion	Hand lotion	Nail polish
Buffing paste	Lemon juice	Nail polish remover
Cleanser	Lip brush	Pumice stone
Cuticle cream	Lip pencil	Razor
Depilatory cream	Lipstick	Salt
Depilatory wax	Manicure stick	10-volume peroxide
Emery boards	Mascara	Toner
Eyeliner	Medicated soap	Waterproof emery
Eye pencils	Medicated talc	paper

Beauty Day 15

Check your hair today. Is it glossier, more manageable? You should see an improvement in its condition if you have been working on the hints given on page 61, Day 7, although getting the oil balance right is only half the story.

Hair takes such a pounding: it's brushed or combed over and over again, exposed to changes of temperature and all sorts of weather conditions. It grows healthy and resistant to damage at scalp level, but becomes progressively more porous towards the ends. On drier, finer hair, the ends split and the infinitesimal cuticles along the hair's surface become roughened when they should be lying flat. This can be improved by using a conditioner after shampooing; but badly damaged hair may look woolly and unkempt until the ends are cut away. With a professional trim every 6 to 8 weeks and regular home care, even the most fragile hair can be kept smooth and shapely.

Choosing your style

There is no point in wearing an ultra-trendy hairstyle if it does nothing for your looks, or aiming for a style which won't suit your hair texture. If hair is fine and straight, it won't naturally take a curly style which needs a lot of body. Perming can add volume to hair and you can read more about this on page 141, Day 17. But the most successful, easy-care style is one where hair is styled to suit its natural texture. For example, fine straight hair worn in a sleek bob with ends cut to shape inwards and under; coarser hair cut to emphasize its natural wave; bushy hair thinned and tapered to keep it under control.

Choosing your stylist

Cutting is something we need to leave to the experts, but there aren't any clear guidelines for finding the right stylist — one who will cut your hair the way you like it.

Personal recommendation is one way. Pluck up courage to ask someone whose style you admire where it originated. Most people enjoy a compliment and will be only too pleased to tell you.

Today's special treatment

Examine the ends of your hair for signs of splitting. View your hair frontwards, in profile and from the back. Does it look shapely from all angles? Could it be time to think about booking an appointment to have your hair reshaped? If so, tick the box below. And if you are 30-plus and you don't intend to tolerate grey hairs, search for them in a strong light. Look carefully at your hairline. Make partings from the centre of your head downwards. Advice for colouring can be found on page 142, Day 17.

Make an appointment to have hair restyled.

Treatment for grey hairs required.

Cleanse, tone, moisturize Cleanse, tone and moisturize your face in the morning and at night.

Hairstyles to choose

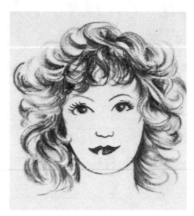

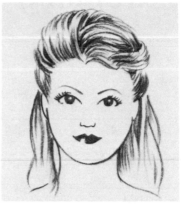

A. *For a long face*
A soft, full style to add
width.

B. *For a round face*
Height to slim. Hair can be
kept longer at the back.

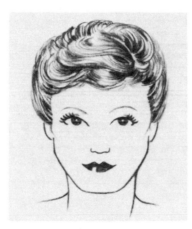

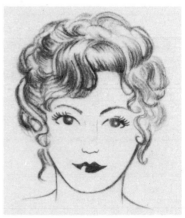

C. *For a square face*
Gentle movement and
height.

D. *For strong features or a
not-so-young face*
Soften with curved sweeps
and strandy curls.

Roughened ankles?	☐	Massage with body cream.
Hair livener	☐	For dry hair only: massage with oil, see page 61, Day 7.
Spotty back?	☐	Soak in warm bath; scrub back with medicated soap, dry and dab with diluted antiseptic. Dust with medicated talc.
Blackheads?	☐	Repeat steam treatment from page 42, Day 4.

Shopping Checklist Day 16

Choose your meals, then write in by each relevant item the amount you require.

Amount required	*Amount required*	*Amount required*
Fruit and Vegetables	**Dairy Produce/Eggs**	Oil-free French dressing
Carrot	Curd cheese	Salt and pepper
Lettuce	Eggs	Stock cube
Mushrooms	Low-fat natural yogurt	Sugar
Onion		Tomato ketchup
Peppers	Low-fat spread	Tomato purée
Potato	Skimmed milk	
Tomatoes	**Grocery**	
Turnip or swede	Bran breakfast cereal	
Apple	Brown rice	
Grapes	Canned tomatoes	
Strawberries or raspberries	Evaporated milk	
Frozen Foods	Instant potato powder	
Broccoli	Low-calorie instant soup	
Strawberries or raspberries	Peanuts	
	Raisins	
Sweetcorn	Sweetcorn	
Vanilla ice cream	Wholemeal bread	
Meat, Poultry and Fish	Wholemeal roll	
Beefburger	**Store Cupboard**	
Beef or pork chipolata sausage	Cornflour	
	Lemon juice	
Streaky bacon	Mixed herbs	
Very lean ground beef	Nutmeg	

Step-by-Step Manicure

Remove old polish one nail at a time. File nails one way only using an emery board. Massage with cuticle cream then soak nails for 5 minutes in water.

Use a basecoat first of all then apply first coat of polish, brushing from cuticle to tip of nail. A second coat of polish gives a long-lasting finish to your manicure.

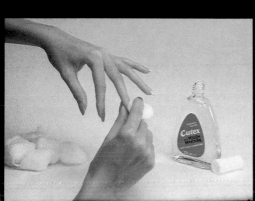
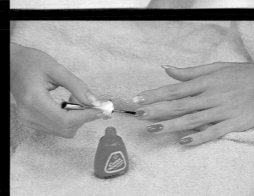

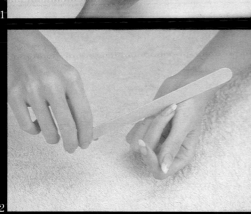
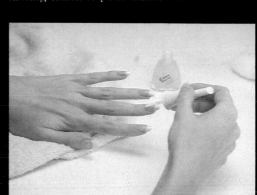

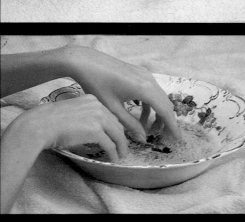
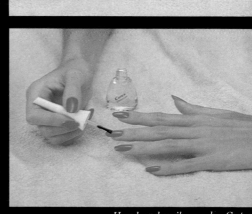

Hand and nail care by Cutex

Changing your hair colour

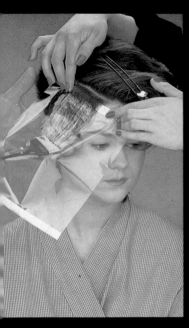

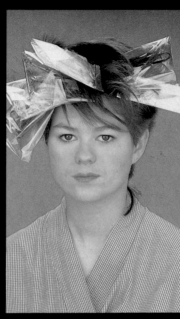

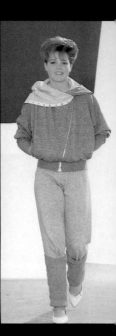

The 'tramming' colour technique can be used to create texture and give volume to hair, but it does need to be done by a professional hairdresser. In the style above

David Blair has used a combination of medium burgundy and soft ash blonde to striking effect.

Semi-permanent colorants that you can use easily at home are usually applied like a shampoo and will last through about six washes. This is the effect you will get with a light auburn colorant if your hair is already light to medium brown or has red highlights.

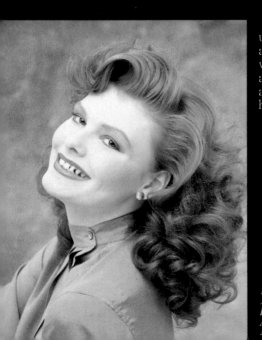

1, 2 and 3: Hair/David Blair, using Wella Koleste 2000 Medium Burgundy and High Lift Soft Ash Blonde. Make-up/Elizabeth Arden. Photography Al Macdonald.
4: Clairol Glints.

Shimmer can shape . . .

If you don't have much lid, take sheen over lids and up to brow — use a light colour such as this silver-blue highlighter.

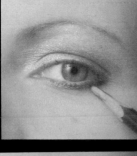

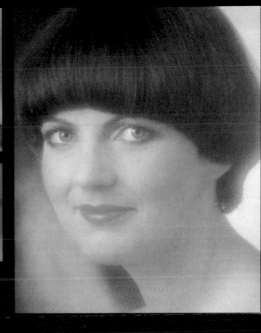

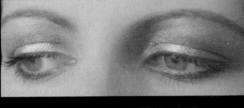

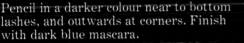

Pencil in a darker colour near to bottom lashes, and outwards at corners. Finish with dark blue mascara.

A super way with silver eyeshadow

With silver on inner lids and smoky grey or navy at outer corners, blend where the colours meet.

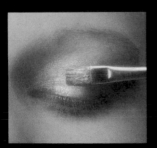

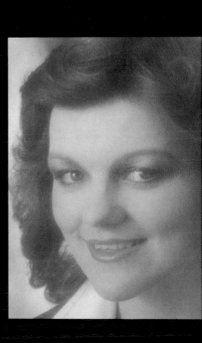

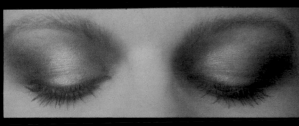

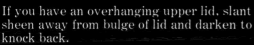

If you have an overhanging upper lid, slant sheen away from bulge of lid and darken to knock back.

Be subtle with sparkle

Gold is a stunning choice for brown eyes.

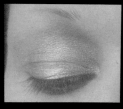 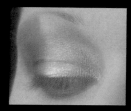

Sweep it over upper lids, with a trace along lower lids close to lashes.

Take a streak of smoky brown from centre lid to brows and close to gold beneath eye.

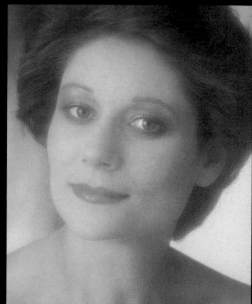

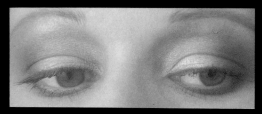

Brush a touch of brown in a curve near nose. Blend brown with gold where the colours meet.
Darker tone at outer corners of eyes makes eyes appear farther apart.

Looking younger . . .

Joan Parsons felt so much younger when she shed over 4st, she wanted to make sure she looked younger, too.

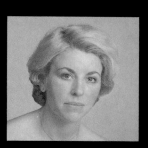

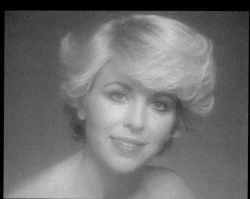

Hair highlighted: a pale ash tone is much softer than an ageing yellow tinge. Hair curving upwards breaks up a hard hairline, gives a lift to face.
Foundation, colour-teamed to palest areas of skin, tones in natural high colour. Avoid using a base that is too pale. It can make you look drawn. Avoid a base that is too dark, it can throw shadows, especially round eyes.
Top with untinted powder, kinder than a shine.

Use a soft grey eye pencil to shade eyes, take colour outwards and slightly upwards at outer corners. Use black or dark brown very finely drawn close to lashes if eyes need more emphasis.
Soft pink lip colour is kind to a full mouth and thin lips.
Soft grey eye pencils used with feathery strokes softens brows. Powdering them lightly first may help. Awfully ageing: thin, over-tweezered brows.

Diet Day 16

☐ *275ml/½ pint skimmed milk or reconstituted low-fat powdered milk*

BREAKFAST/SUPPER MEAL

Either ☐ *2 tomatoes, grilled without fat; 2 beef or pork chipolata sausages well grilled; 1 small slice wholemeal bread, 25g/1oz*

Or ☐ *1 egg, size 3, boiled; 1 small slice wholemeal bread, 25g/1oz; 5ml/1 level teaspoon low-fat spread*

Or ☐ *25g/1oz any bran breakfast cereal; 60ml/4 level tablespoons low-fat natural yogurt; 6 grapes*

LIGHT MEAL

Either to eat at home
Vegetable Soup and Bread
☐
50g/2oz turnip or swede
1 small carrot
1 small onion
115g/4oz potato
2 tomatoes
200ml/7floz stock, made with ½ stock cube

Salt and pepper
10ml/2 level teaspoons tomato purée
1 small slice wholemeal bread, 25g/1oz

Dice turnip or swede, carrot, onion and potato. Chop tomatoes. Put vegetables in a saucepan with stock, seasoning and tomato purée and bring to the boil. Cover and simmer for 30 minutes. Serve soup with bread.

Or to take to work
Soup, Salad Roll plus Fruit
☐
1 sachet low-calorie instant soup, any flavour
1 wholemeal bread roll, 50g/2oz

25g/1oz curd cheese
Lettuce
Tomato
1 small apple

Make up soup at work or take to work in a vacuum flask. Cut roll in half and spread both sides with curd cheese. Fill with as much lettuce and tomato slices as you wish. Take apple to eat after roll.

Either a quick recipe
Eggburger and Vegetables plus Berries and Ice Cream

1 beefburger, 50g/2oz raw
45ml/3 level tablespoons
  instant potato powder
1 egg, size 3
115g/4oz broccoli

115g/4oz strawberries or
  raspberries, fresh or
  frozen
50g/2oz vanilla ice cream

Grill beefburger well. Make up the instant potato powder and spoon around cooked burger. Poach egg in a little water or non-stick poacher without fat and place on top of burger. Boil broccoli and serve with eggburger. Follow with berries and ice cream.

Or a keen cook's recipe
Shepherd's Pie and Vegetables plus Apple Whip

75g/3oz very lean ground
  beef
1 small onion
50g/2oz mushrooms
Half 200g/7oz can tomatoes
Salt and pepper
Pinch mixed herbs
60ml/4 tablespoons stock
  made with stock cube
10ml/2 level teaspoons
  cornflour

150g/5oz potato
15ml/1 tablespoon skimmed
  milk
115g/4oz broccoli
1 medium apple
5ml/1 teaspoon lemon juice
5ml/1 level teaspoon sugar
30ml/2 tablespoons
  evaporated milk
Pinch nutmeg

Put meat into a small non-stick pan and heat gently, stirring for 5-10 minutes. Drain off any fat. Finely chop onion, slice mushrooms and add to pan with tomatoes and seasonings. Add stock and juice from tomatoes, cover and simmer for about 30 minutes. Mix cornflour with a little cold water until smooth and add to meat. Boil until thickened. Boil potato and mash with skimmed milk. Transfer meat to a small ovenproof dish and spread potato on top. Grill to brown and serve with broccoli. To follow: peel, core and chop apple and put into a blender with lemon juice, sugar, evaporated milk and nutmeg. Blend until smooth and pour into a dish.

Or if you prefer to eat vegetarian
Fiesta Salad plus Yogurt

115g/4oz sweetcorn, canned
  or frozen
25g/1oz brown rice
Salt
½ red or green pepper

25g/1oz dry roasted peanuts
30ml/2 tablespoons oil-free
  French dressing
1 small carton low-fat natural
  yogurt

Cook frozen sweetcorn or drain canned corn. Cook rice in boiling, salted water; drain and rinse in cold water. Discard stem and seeds from peppers and chop flesh. Add peppers to sweetcorn with peanuts, rice and dressing. Mix well. Follow with yogurt.

Snack 1 ☐ *30ml/2 level tablespoons*   *15ml/1 level tablespoon*
     raisins   *peanuts*

Snack 2 ☐ *2 rashers streaky bacon, well*   *2 small slices wholemeal*
     grilled   *bread, 25g/1oz each*
     15ml/1 tablespoon tomato
     ketchup

☐ If you completed the day without cheating at all, tick here and move on to Day 17.

☐ If you cheated, do a 'Saintly Day' tomorrow (page 253) instead of the set menu.

☐ If you do not eat one meal or snack that you are allowed, tick this box and save up for a 'Naughty Day'. When you have two ticks saved, you can do any of the Thoroughly Naughty Day's Menus *instead* of your next day's diet.

Exercise Day 16

MORNING ☐ Repeat Exercise 1: 5 times

☐ Repeat Exercise 2: 5 times to right
5 times to left

☐ Repeat Exercise 3: 5 times circling left and right with right foot
5 times circling left and right with left foot

☐ Repeat Exercise 4: touch the floor 15 times

☐ Repeat Exercise 5: bend to the left and right 15 times

☐ Repeat Exercise 6: circle to left 15 times
circle to right 15 times

☐ Repeat Exercise 7: criss-cross 20 times

☐ Repeat Exercise 8: stretch 5 times

☐ Repeat Exercise 9: touch left foot and sit up
touch right foot and sit up 10 times

LUNCHTIME ☐ Walk for 20 minutes. Turn and return the same way in 16 minutes.

EVENING ☐ Run to the top of the stairs and down again 4 times. Jog for 10 minutes.

Or ☐ Jog for 17 minutes:
1st 5-minute jog
2nd 5-minute jog
3rd 5-minute jog
4th 2-minute jog

You will need a skipping rope for tomorrow's exercises. A piece of washing line will do.

Bedtime Relaxer ☐

Beauty Day 16

Considering that it takes around 6 months for a new nail to grow from root to fingertip, a broken or split nail can be made to look respectable in a very short time. File the rough edge lightly, and within a few days a white rim appears at the nail tip and the nail will look longer.

Only very strong nails are proof against breakage, and the strength or frailty of nails is something you inherit. Weak nails can be strengthened but they need continuous care. Polish by rubbing backwards and forwards across the palm of your hand whenever you use hand cream, and manicure to improve the appearance of the shortest nails. Have you tried the treatment we suggested on page 54, Day 6?

Can nail polish help?
It protects weak nails and gives them a temporary toughness, which therefore makes them less vulnerable to damage. They look more cared-for with the gloss that polish gives them, although for stubby nails a pale or colourless

shade draws less attention than a bolder tone.

A base coat can be a good beauty investment. Apply before using coloured polish. It acts as an 'undercoat', makes top polish more durable and provides a smooth surface by glossing over dents and ridges. Those ridges tell a story. The horizontal kind may reflect recent ill-health. Ridges which run vertically are evidence of pressure having been exerted on the nail bed while the nail was soft and still forming. So are tiny white flecks, which eventually grow out. A vertical ridge may become a permanent feature but try painting extra coats of nail polish either side.

A professional polish takes time. It needs patience and practice and it is a mistake to apply polish too thickly because it then takes a long time to dry. Watch a well-trained manicurist. She uses the minimum of polish, applying it in thin coats, allowing each to dry before the next is applied.

When nail polish chips at the edges retouch with a tiny slick of polish on the bared section. When this dries, apply polish along the length of the nail.

Choosing your colour
Trends apart, basic rules apply. Paler shades do more than dark moody tones to make hands and nails appear longer and slimmer. Colours which reflect skin tone look more elegant than those that clash with it. Choose pink polish or rosy red if skin has a natural pink tinge, chestnut or coral if it is sallow or tanned.

* Keep polish in the refrigerator. It's easier to apply and dries more quickly when chilled.

* Keep the bottle top free of polish so that you won't have to wrench the cap to remove it next time. Loosen hardened polish with cotton wool dabbed with remover, but take care it doesn't remove the polish from your nails.

Today's special treatment:
Repeat manicure, see page 54, Day 6, then apply polish as follows:

1. Stroke the brush on the inside of the bottle to remove surplus polish. You should be able to hold up the brush without it dripping.

2. Paint a stripe in the centre of the nail, from cuticle to tip.

3. Paint either side of this stripe, flexing brush lightly to spread the colour to the outer corners of the nail.

☐ 4. Allow nails to dry for 10 minutes before applying a second coat of polish.

Nails bitten short? ☐ Colourless polish improves their looks.

Spotty back? ☐ Soak in warm bath; scrub back with medicated soap, dry and dab with diluted antiseptic. Dust with medicated talc.

Body massage ☐ Repeat the body massage from page 29, Day 2.

Cleanse, tone, moisturize ☐ Cleanse, tone and moisturize your face in the morning and at night.

Hair livener ☐ Massage scalp, see page 61, Day 7, but omit oil.

Shopping Checklist Day 17

Choose your meals, then write in by each relevant item the amount you require.

Amount required	*Amount required*	*Amount required*
Fruit and Vegetables	**Meat, Poultry and Fish**	**Store Cupboard**
Brussels sprouts	Chicken	Chicken stock cube
Carrots	Mussels	Cornflour
Chives	Prawns	Jam
Leek	Streaky bacon	Marmalade
Onion	**Dairy Produce/Eggs**	Nutmeg
Potato	Cheddar cheese	Oil-free French
Swede	Double Gloucester or	dressing
Tomato	Stilton cheese	Salt and pepper
Apple	Eggs	
Banana	Low-fat natural	
Pear	yogurt	
Raspberries or	Low-fat spread	
strawberries	Skimmed milk	
Frozen Foods	**Grocery**	
Brussels sprouts	Bran breakfast cereal	
Peas and baby carrots	Cream crackers	
Raspberries or	Creamed rice pudding	
strawberries	Dried apricots	
Rice, peas	Lemon juice	
and mushrooms	Onion sauce mix	
Rice, sweetcorn and	Prunes	
peppers	Skimmed milk powder	
Spinach	Wholemeal bread	
Swede	Wholemeal roll	

Diet Day 17

☐ 275ml/½ pint skimmed milk or reconstituted low-fat powdered milk

BREAKFAST/SUPPER MEAL

Either ☐ 2 eggs, size 3, scrambled with 15ml/1 tablespoon skimmed milk (extra to allowance); 1 tomato, grilled without fat

Or ☐ 25g/1oz any bran breakfast cereal; 75ml/5 tablespoons skimmed milk; 2 dried apricots, chopped

Or ☐ 2 small slices wholemeal bread, 25g/1oz each, toasted; 10ml/2 level teaspoons low-fat spread; 10ml/2 level teaspoons marmalade or jam

LIGHT MEAL

Either to eat at home
Paella plus Apple

☐ Half 227g/8oz packet frozen rice, peas and mushrooms
50g/2oz shelled prawns, fresh, frozen or canned
50g/2oz shelled mussels
1 small apple

Cook rice and vegetables as instructed on packet. Add prawns and mussels and warm through. Follow with apple.

Or to take to work
Prawn and Rice Salad plus Banana

☐ Half 227g/8oz packet frozen rice, sweetcorn and peppers
50g/2oz shelled prawns
15ml/1 tablespoon oil-free French dressing
1 medium banana

Cook rice and vegetables as instructed and allow to cool. Mix with prawns and French dressing and take to work in a plastic container. Follow with banana.

Or if you prefer to eat vegetarian
Spinach Soup and Roll

☐ 115g/4oz chopped spinach, frozen
25g/1oz onion
150ml/¼ pint water
¼ chicken stock cube
30ml/2 level tablespoons skimmed milk powder
10ml/2 level teaspoons cornflour
2.5ml/½ level teaspoon lemon juice
Pinch nutmeg
30ml/2 level tablespoons low-fat natural yogurt
1 wholemeal roll, 50g/2oz

Defrost spinach. Finely chop onion and place in a small saucepan with water and stock cube. Bring to boil, cover and simmer for 10 minutes. Blend skimmed milk powder and cornflour with a little cold water and add to saucepan, stirring until mixture thickens. Add spinach, lemon juice and nutmeg; stir. Simmer for 5 minutes. For a smoother soup, liquidize then return to pan and reheat. Swirl in yogurt before serving with wholemeal roll. Soup can be taken to work in a flask and yogurt omitted.

MAIN MEAL

Either a
quick recipe
Chicken and
Vegetables
plus Berries

75g/3oz cooked chicken meat
150g/6oz potato
45ml/3 level tablespoons
  low-fat natural yogurt
Chives, optional
115g/4oz Brussels sprouts,
  fresh or frozen

115g/4oz swede or carrots,
  fresh or frozen
115g/4oz raspberries or
  strawberries, fresh or
  frozen

Remove any skin or fat from chicken and cut into slices. Bake scrubbed potato in its jacket at 200°C/400°F, gas mark 6, for about 40 minutes or until soft when pinched. Top with 15ml/1 level tablespoon yogurt and chives. (The stuffed potato can be prepared the night before and kept in the refrigerator. When you are ready to use, reheat in oven for about 15 minutes.) Serve carrots, or swede mashed with a little pepper, with sprouts, baked potato and chicken. Follow with berries topped with remaining yogurt.

Or a keen
cook's recipe
Prune-Stuffed
Chicken plus
Berries

4 dried or ready-to-eat
  prunes
150g/5oz boned chicken
  breast, raw
½ small onion
1 rasher streaky bacon
60ml/4 level tablespoons
  fresh breadcrumbs
Salt and pepper

75g/3oz swede or carrots,
  fresh or frozen
75g/3oz Brussels sprouts,
  fresh or frozen
115g/4oz raspberries or
  strawberries
30ml/2 level tablespoons low-
  fat natural yogurt

Soak dried prunes overnight in water. Discard skin then place the chicken between two pieces of greaseproof paper and beat until thin. Drain and stone dried prunes and cut them into small pieces. Chop onion; boil for about 5 minutes and drain. Grill the bacon well and chop. Mix together the onion, bacon, prunes, breadcrumbs and seasoning. Spread chicken breast with stuffing mixture and fold over. Tie with string or secure with wooden cocktail stick. Wrap chicken in foil and bake at 180°C/350°F gas mark 4, for 1 hour.

Serve carrots, or swede mashed with a little pepper, with sprouts and stuffed chicken. Follow with berries topped with yogurt.

Or if you prefer to eat vegetarian **Cheese and Onion Medley plus Pear**

50g/2oz white part of leek	*Salt and pepper*
225g/8oz peas and baby carrots, frozen	*25g/1oz Cheddar cheese*
½ packet onion sauce mix	*25g/1oz fresh wholemeal breadcrumbs*
150ml/¼ pint skimmed milk	*1 pear*

Slice leek and place in a pan of boiling water along with peas and carrots. Cook until all vegetables are tender. Make up onion sauce using skimmed milk. Add drained vegetables and warm through. Season and turn into an ovenproof dish. Grate cheese, mix with breadcrumbs and sprinkle over top of vegetables. Grill until cheese melts. Follow with pear.

Snack 1

25g/1oz Cheddar, Double Gloucester or Stilton cheese	*2 cream crackers*
	1 medium apple

Snack 2

170g/6oz can creamed rice pudding	*10ml/2 level teaspoons jam*
	1 medium apple

If you completed the day without cheating at all, tick here and move on to Day 18.

If you cheated, do a 'Saintly Day' tomorrow (page 253) instead of the set menu.

If you do not eat one meal or snack that you are allowed, tick this box and save up for a 'Naughty Day'. When you have two ticks saved, you can do any of the Thoroughly Naughty Day's Menus *instead* of your next day's diet.

Exercise Day 17

MORNING ☐ Repeat Exercise 1: 5 times

☐ Repeat Exercise 2: 5 times to right
5 times to left

☐ Repeat Exercise 3: 5 times circling left and right with right foot
5 times circling left and right with left foot

☐ Repeat Exercise 4: touch floor 15 times

☐ Repeat Exercise 5: bend to the left and right 15 times

☐ Repeat Exercise 6: circle to left 15 times
circle to right 15 times

☐ Repeat Exercise 7: criss-cross 20 times

☐ Repeat Exercise 8: stretch 5 times

☐ Repeat Exercise 9: touch left foot and sit up
touch right foot and sit up 15 times
Keep those legs straight as you bend forwards. You may not be able to reach your foot at first, but you will probably find that you are able to reach a little further down your leg each time you repeat the exercise.

LUNCHTIME ☐ Walk for 21 minutes. Turn and return the same way in 17 minutes.

EVENING ☐ Run to the top of the stairs and down again 4 times. Jog for 10 minutes.

Or ☐ Jog for 17 minutes:
1st 5-minute jog
2nd 5-minute jog
3rd 5-minute jog
4th 2-minute jog

Then skip as follows ☐ Start with feet together and rope behind feet. Swing the rope up over your head and jump over rope as you bring it down to the floor before you. Land first on the left foot and then on the right foot in a jogging movement. Do 25 skips.

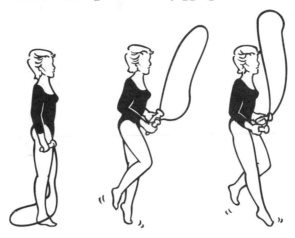

Bedtime Relaxer ☐

Beauty Day 17

Perming

If your hair is hard to manage, a perm could help. Your regular hairdresser will have a fair idea of whether your hair is suitable for perming. Some hair 'takes' very well, but other hair is resistant to perming, and very fine hair can frizz. If you are in doubt, ask your hairdresser to do a trial strand of hair where it won't show. Perms act by changing the chemical structure of the hair. The hair is wound around curlers and softened with one type of lotion. The curl is then 'fixed' with another lotion. Much depends on the strength of the perming lotions, the built-in conditioners, the skill of the hairdresser, and the health and texture of your hair. Hair should be cut and shaped before perming; and, especially if you have never had a perm before, it is best to have it done by professionals rather than attempt a home-perm. A successful perm gives hair extra body, adds soft movement or curl to straight hair and leaves it shiny and supple. Today's perms can be very light, just giving the hair extra body, or can produce tight curls. Talk to your hairdresser about the sort of style you are aiming for and he/she will advise on the strength of perm required.

It is important to make sure that your hair is in good condition before you have a perm. Dry and porous hair can be over-processed and perming could dry it even more. A perm will last until it grows out, so it is worth while buying the best you can afford. A cut-price offer can mean an inferior product or a rushed service. Tell the stylist if you have used a colorant on your hair, for this can affect how the perm takes. Always condition your hair well after having a perm. If you want to colour your hair (see below), remember that your hair is likely to be extra porous after a perm and will therefore require a shorter colouring time.

Colouring
Colorants for hair are usually labelled permanent, semi-permanent or temporary. The permanent kind can change hair colour completely. The colour won't wash out, although it may fade a little. Semi-permanent colorants last through, perhaps, half a dozen shampoos (the packet will tell you how many). The temporaries wash out and add a light wash of colour or highlights to hair. If a colorant isn't clearly marked permanent, then identify it by the label: 'lasting colour'. Two substances which have to be mixed together before using will usually produce permanent colouring.

Most products which claim to lighten hair have a permanent effect. Hair which is naturally dark blonde, mousy or light brown can look stunning when it's bleached blonde all over or streaked with sunlit highlights. Highlighting, though, takes expertise and is best left to professional hairdressers. There may be problems when dark hair is lightened and it is worth paying for professional advice. Lightened hair will not always blend with dark skin tones, and the natural pigment in dark hair can produce a 'brassy' tinge. Eyebrows could need bleaching, too.

When colour is 'semi-permanent' it adds darker, richer colour, warmer brown or red tones, or blonde highlights to fair hair. It disguises a sprinkling of grey hairs but more extensive grey hair may need to be professionally coloured. A blue rinse will give naturally grey hair a more silvery tone.

Today's special treatment
Feet should be ready for another pedicure. Step-by-step details can be found on page 81, Day 9.

Check for regrowth of unwanted hair because if you can see it, so can others. See page 86, Day 10.

Cleanse, tone, moisturize	☐	Cleanse, tone and moisturize your face in the morning and at night.
Hair livener	☐	For dry hair only: massage scalp, see page 61, Day 7, but omit oil.
Elbows	☐	Still rough or discoloured? Mix lemon juice with a little salt and rub in. Rinse off after 5 to 10 minutes and apply body lotion.
Dinginess?	☐	Blend hand cream with 6 drops of 10-volume peroxide and smooth it into dingy areas on thighs and under arms.
Goosepimples?	☐	Lather goosepimply areas with a soft brush. Splash with cold water, pat dry and rub in cream or body lotion.
Roughened ankles?	☐	Massage with body cream.
Spotty back?	☐	Soak in warm bath; scrub back with medicated soap, dry and dab with diluted antiseptic. Dust with medicated talc.
Neck treatment	☐	Repeat treatment on page 49, Day 5, to keep neck supple.

Shopping Checklist Day 18

Choose your meals, then write in by each relevant item the amount you require.

Amount required	Amount required	Amount required
Fruit and Vegetables	Low-fat natural	Salt and pepper
Carrot	yogurt	Sherry
Cauliflower	Low-fat spread	Soy sauce
Celery	Skimmed milk	Tomato ketchup
Green cabbage	**Grocery**	Worcestershire sauce
Green pepper	Baked beans in	
Onion	tomato sauce	
Tomato	Bran breakfast cereal	
Watercress	Brown rice	
Apple	Crispbreads	
Banana	Curry sauce mix	
Grapefruit	French bread	
Orange	Jelly*	
Frozen Foods	Liver pâté	
Sweetcorn	Pasta shells	
Meat, Poultry and Fish	Raisins or sultanas	
Chicken	Sweetcorn	
Lamb loin chop	Wholemeal bread	
Leg of lamb	**Store Cupboard**	
Streaky bacon	Artificial sweetener	
Dairy Produce/Eggs	Bay leaf	
Cottage cheese	Brown sugar	
Edam or Tendale	Curry paste	
cheese	Low-calorie salad	
Eggs	dressing	

*Jelly will need to be made in advance to allow time for setting.

Diet Day 18

☐ 275ml/½ pint skimmed milk or reconstituted low-fat powdered milk

BREAKFAST/SUPPER MEAL

Either ☐ 1 slice wholemeal bread, 40g/1½oz; 1 egg, size 3; 5ml/1 level teaspoon low-fat spread
Dip bread in beaten egg and fry in a non-stick pan greased with low-fat spread.

Or ☐ 25g/1oz any bran breakfast cereal; 60ml/4 level tablespoons low-fat natural yogurt; 15ml/1 level tablespoon raisins or sultanas

Or ☐ 2 rashers streaky bacon; 2 tomatoes; 1 small slice wholemeal bread, 25g/1oz

LIGHT MEAL

Either to eat at home
Chicken Curry and Rice plus Grapefruit

☐ 50g/2oz cooked chicken meat 25g/1oz brown rice, raw
½ packet curry sauce mix   ½ grapefruit
Remove any skin or fat from chicken and cut meat into cubes. Make up curry sauce mix as instructed on packet and add chicken. Serve with boiled rice. The grapefruit can be eaten before or after the chicken curry.

Or to take to work
Chicken Curry Salad plus Fruit

☐ 75g/3oz carrot   5ml-10ml/1-2 level teaspoons
15ml/1 level tablespoon   curry paste
   raisins   50g/2oz cooked chicken meat
Watercress   1 small banana
30ml/2 tablespoons low-   ½ grapefruit
   calorie salad dressing
Grate carrot and mix with raisins and chopped watercress. Place in the bottom of a container. Mix together salad dressing and curry paste and fold in cubed chicken (any skin or fat removed). Place on top of salad. Slice banana and mix with grapefruit. Take to work in a separate container.

Or if you prefer to eat vegetarian
Cheese and Egg Crispbreads

☐ 1 egg, size 3   .4 crispbreads
113g/4oz carton cottage cheese,
   natural or with chives

145

Hard boil the egg; cool, shell and chop. Mix egg with cottage cheese and serve with crispbreads.

MAIN MEAL

Either a quick recipe **Lamb Chop and Vegetables plus Fruit Jelly**

150g/5oz lamb loin chop
115g/4oz cauliflower
115g/4oz green cabbage
30ml/2 level tablespoons tomato ketchup

¼ jelly, any flavour
115ml/¼ pint boiling water
½ grapefruit
1 medium orange

Discard all visible fat and well grill the lamb chop. Boil cauliflower and cabbage. Gently heat ketchup and serve over chop accompanied by vegetables. Make up jelly with boiling water and allow to cool. Peel and segment grapefruit and orange and add to jelly. Allow to set and eat after main course.

Or a keen cook's recipe **Lamb Kebab with Pasta plus Grilled Grapefruit**

50g/2oz leg of lamb
1 small onion
½ green pepper
1 bay leaf
45ml/3 tablespoons tomato ketchup
5ml/1 teaspoon Soy sauce
5ml/1 teaspoon Worcestershire sauce

25g/1oz pasta shells, raw
50g/2oz sweetcorn, frozen or canned
½ grapefruit
15ml/1 tablespoon sherry
10ml/2 level teaspoons brown sugar

Discard all fat then cut meat into cubes. Boil onion whole for about 10 minutes, then quarter. Cut pepper into 8 pieces. Thread meat, onion and pepper onto a kebab stick or skewer, with the bay leaf. Mix together tomato ketchup, Soy sauce and Worcestershire sauce. Spread a little on the kebab and grill for about 12 minutes, turning occasionally. Serve any remaining sauce separately. Boil pasta shells and sweetcorn and serve with kebab. Loosen grapefruit segments but keep in shell. Sprinkle with sherry and top with sugar. Grill until sugar melts, then serve.

Of if you prefer to eat vegetarian **Beans and Cheese Medley**

225g/7.9oz can baked beans in tomato sauce
1 stick celery
¼ green pepper
50g/2oz cauliflower

25g/1oz Edam or Tendale cheese
2 slices wholemeal bread, 25g/1oz each

Place beans in a small saucepan and heat gently. Chop celery and green pepper; cut cauliflower in small florets. Add vegetables to pan and heat through. Stir in cubed cheese. Serve on toasted bread.

Snack 1 ☐   *50g/2oz slice French bread*   *40g/1½oz liver pâté*

Snack 2 ☐   *1 small carton low-fat*   *1 large banana*
               natural yogurt   *1 medium apple*
Either eat individually or cut up fruit and mix with yogurt.

☐   If you completed the day without cheating at all, tick here and move on to Day 19.

☐   If you cheated, do a 'Saintly Day' tomorrow (page 253) instead of the set menu.

☐   If you do not eat one meal or snack that you are allowed, tick this box and save up for a 'Naughty Day'.
When you have two ticks saved, you can do any of the Thoroughly Naughty Day's Menus *instead* of your next day's diet.

Exercise Day 18

MORNING ☐   Repeat Exercise 1: 5 times

☐   Repeat Exercise 2: 5 times to right
6 times to left

☐   Repeat Exercise 3: 5 times circling left and right with right foot
5 times circling left and right with left foot

☐   Repeat Exercise 4: touch the floor 15 times

☐   Repeat Exercise 5: bend to the left and right 15 times

☐   Repeat Exercise 6: circle to left 15 times
circle to right 15 times

☐   Repeat Exercise 7: criss-cross 20 times

☐   Repeat Exercise 8: stretch 5 times

☐ Repeat Exercise 9: touch left foot and sit up
touch right foot and sit up 15 times

Exercise 10 ☐ Sit with legs in front of you.
Move forward, walking on
your bottom, swinging your
arms backwards and
forwards to help you move
your body along. When you
come within inches of a wall,
go into reverse and floor-
walk backwards.

LUNCHTIME ☐ Walk for 22 minutes but this time mark your position 2
minutes from your starting point. Turn and briskly return
to your marked place in 15 minutes, then jog the final
stretch.
*If you find you are embarrassed to be seen jogging around
at lunchtime you could save your 2-minute jog for the
evening. Or do it first thing in the morning.*

EVENING ☐ Run to the top of the stairs and down again 4 times. Jog for
10 minutes.

Or ☐ Jog for 18 minutes:
1st 5-minute jog
2nd 5-minute jog
3rd 5-minute jog
4th 3-minute jog

Then ☐ Skip 50 times.

Bedtime Relaxer ☐

Beauty Day 18

Make-up
Make-up can work wonders if it's used in the right way,
emphasizing your best features. It can also help to protect
your skin against the elements. Foundation acts as a barrier
against drying wind and grime, as well as adding a pretty
film of colour to your skin.

It is easy to make a mistake when choosing foundation. That's partly because there is such a wide choice; everything from light liquids to cover-up cake formulas. So how can you find the right one for you?

Start with texture
Most foundations come in several shades, but concentrate first of all on getting the texture right. The idea, of course, is not to look 'made-up'. There is no point in covering up a fresh, clear skin with a heavy foundation but a light, see-through fluid can add a soft sheen of colour.

Oily skin
For oily skin there are light fluid foundations which are powder-based. They won't add oil; they help absorb it. Look for 'matt' or 'oil-free' on the label. It is very important to cleanse your skin and use an astringent toning lotion before applying your foundation.

Dry skin
For dry skin there are fluid bases which are a little oilier. The label gives you a clue by mentioning 'moisturized' or 'richer'. Cream foundations are normally geared towards dry skin but there are exceptions, so check the manufacturer's recommendations. Always apply a lavish amount of moisturizer to a dry skin before using foundation.

Combination skin
A combination skin with an oily centre panel can be classed as oily for make-up purposes; but treat the dry areas to moisturizer before using foundation.

Choosing foundation colour
Names and shade cards help, but insist on testing a foundation before choosing. Colours may look different on your skin than in a bottle. Smooth a little foundation on the inside of your wrist where the skin is similar in texture and tone to that on your face. Match your skin tone or, when in doubt, choose a cool beige. Foundation 'warms' on some skin and any extra colour you need can come from using blusher.

Here's how to apply foundation
Use fingertips to apply light creams and liquids. Dot a blob on cheeks, forehead, nose and chin. Use light strokes upwards and outwards from cheeks to temples. Stroke downwards over forehead, working outwards to temples. Blend outwards over cheeks and down nose, carefully

around nostrils. Downward on upper lip and upwards from centre of chin. Stroke away the colour round chinline to avoid any tide-mark. Do not rub foundation into skin or use too much. The idea is to cover your face with a light film.

Face powder
Make-up will last much longer if you powder on top of your foundation. Use translucent untinted powder which won't add colour. Fluff over face with a piece of cotton wool, then stroke downwards with cotton wool or powder brush to remove surplus.

Applying blusher
Blusher adds colour but it can also be used to shape. Choose creamy blusher if you have a dry skin or prefer not to powder. Apply it after your foundation, just below cheekbones. Use powder blusher after powdering. Fluff powder on with a broad brush which can be bought separately if it is not included with your blusher. Try a touch of blusher on chin or over forehead to liven your colouring. When using blusher to shape face (see illustration) remember that a dark colour will 'thin' an area, while a light colour will emphasize it. Blusher should tone with your lipstick colour.

Blusher can be used to shape as well as to colour. Here it's brushed inwards from outer cheeks to 'slim' a round face.

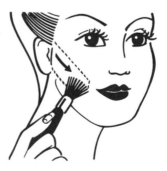

Today's special treatment
Repeat the home facial from page 37, Day 3. You may have discovered it brings up your colour because it stimulates circulation. So wait at least an hour before applying make-up.

Cleanse, tone, moisturize

Cleanse, tone and moisturize your face in the morning and at night.

Hair livener

Massage scalp, see page 61, Day 7, but omit oil.

Roughened ankles? ☐ Massage with body cream.

Blackheads? ☐ Repeat steam treatment from page 42, Day 4.

Shopping Checklist Day 19

Choose your meals, then write in by each relevant item the amount you require.

Amount required	Amount required	Amount required
Fruit and Vegetables	**Dairy Produce/Eggs**	**Store Cupboard**
Bean sprouts	Cottage cheese	Low-calorie seafood
Carrot	Edam or Tendale	or tartare sauce
Celery	cheese	Mixed herbs
Courgettes	Eggs	Salt and pepper
Garlic	Low-fat natural	Soy sauce
Green cabbage	yogurt	Stock cube
Green pepper	Low-fat spread	Vinegar
Leek	Skimmed milk	
Mushrooms	Whole milk	
Mustard and cress	**Grocery**	
Onion	Baked beans in	
Potato	tomato sauce	
Tomatoes	Bean sprouts	
Watercress	Bran breakfast cereal	
Peach	Brown rice	
Pear	Chocolate-flavour	
Frozen Foods	sauce	
Courgettes	Coffee essence	
Vanilla ice cream	Digestive biscuits	
Meat, Poultry and Fish	Liver pâté	
Cod steaks	Low-calorie soup	
Cod steak in	Pineapple canned	
breadcrumbs	in natural juice	
Streaky bacon	Raisins or sultanas	
	Wholemeal bread	

Diet Day 19

☐ *275ml/½ pint skimmed milk or reconstituted low-fat powdered milk*

Either ☐ *2 tomatoes, grilled without fat; 2 rashers streaky bacon, well grilled; 1 small slice wholemeal bread, 25g/1oz*

Or ☐ *1 egg, size 3, boiled; 1 small slice wholemeal bread, 25g/1oz; 5ml/1 level teaspoon low-fat spread*

Or ☐ *25g/1oz any bran breakfast cereal; 75ml/5 tablespoons skimmed milk (extra to allowance); 15ml/1 level tablespoon raisins or sultanas*

LIGHT MEAL

Either to eat at home **Minestrone Soup plus Bread**

☐

50g/2oz baked beans in tomato sauce	*½ stock cube*
1 stick celery	*Pinch mixed herbs*
1 small onion	*Salt and pepper*
1 small carrot	*25g/1oz Edam or Tendale cheese*
3 tomatoes	*1 small slice wholemeal bread, 25g/1oz*
50g/2oz green cabbage	
275ml/½ pint boiling water	

Put beans in a saucepan with sliced celery, chopped onion, diced carrot, chopped tomatoes and finely shredded cabbage. Add herbs and seasoning, boiling water, stock cube. Bring to the boil, cover and simmer for 15 minutes. Grate cheese and sprinkle over soup. Serve with bread.

Or to take to work **Soup plus Cheese and Cress Sandwich**

☐

1 sachet instant low-calorie soup, any flavour	*50g/2oz cottage cheese*
2 small slices wholemeal bread, 25g/1oz each	*Mustard and cress or watercress*

Take sachet of soup to work and mix with hot water or take mixed soup to work in a flask. Make a sandwich with bread, cottage cheese and cress and eat after soup.

Either a quick recipe **Cod Steak in Breadcrumbs plus Ice Cream**

1 frozen cod steak in breadcrumbs, 100g/3½oz
150g/5oz potato
15ml/1 tablespoon skimmed milk

115g/4oz courgettes, fresh or frozen
2 tomatoes
15ml/1 tablespoon low-calorie seafood or tartare sauce
50g/2oz vanilla ice cream

Grill cod steak without adding fat. Boil potato, then mash with milk. Boil sliced courgettes and grill the tomato without adding fat. Serve cod steak with vegetables and seafood or tartare sauce. Follow with ice cream.

Or a keen cook's recipe **Baked Cod with Vegetables plus Pear Sundae**

2 cod steaks, fresh or frozen, 100g/3½oz each
1 rasher streaky bacon
1 leek or small onion
1 courgette
2 tomatoes
Salt and pepper

30ml/2 tablespoons stock made with stock cube
115g/4oz bean sprouts, fresh or canned
25g/1oz vanilla ice cream
15ml/1 tablespoon chocolate-flavour sauce
1 small pear or peach

There is no need to defrost cod steaks before baking, but if they are frozen add 15 minutes to cooking time. Grill the bacon well, discarding any fat that cooks out. Boil thinly sliced leek and sliced courgette for about 10 minutes and drain. Put vegetables at the bottom of an ovenproof dish and place cod steaks on top. Season and top with chopped bacon and tomato slices. Pour over stock, cover with lid or foil and bake at 190°C/375°F gas mark 5, for 30 minutes. Serve with lightly boiled bean sprouts. Peel and halve pear or peach and top with ice cream. Pour chocolate sauce over ice cream and serve immediately.

Or if you prefer to eat vegetarian **Chinese Style Rice plus Coffee Ice Cream**

25g/1oz brown rice
25g/1oz onion
¼ green pepper
1 ring pineapple canned in natural juice
50g/2oz mushrooms
½ clove garlic
1 egg, size 3
10ml/2 level teaspoons low-fat spread

50g/2oz bean sprouts, fresh or frozen
2.5ml/½ teaspoon Soy sauce
2.5ml/½ teaspoon vinegar
60ml/4 level tablespoons low-fat natural yogurt
5ml/1 teaspoon coffee essence
15g/½oz raisins
25g/1oz vanilla ice cream

Cook rice in boiling salted water for about 40 minutes or until cooked. Chop onion, pepper, pineapple and mushrooms. Crush garlic. Lightly beat egg. Brush 5ml/1 level teaspoon low-fat spread over surface of non-stick pan;

pour in egg and make an omelet. Remove omelet and keep warm. Drain cooked rice and keep warm. Melt remaining low-fat spread in the frying pan; add prepared vegetables, garlic and bean sprouts. Stir briskly for 2-3 minutes. Mix together Soy sauce and vinegar; add to vegetables and cooked rice. Heat through, stirring. Cut omelet into strips; stir into rice and vegetable mixture. Serve immediately. Blend together yogurt and coffee essence then stir in raisins. Serve ice cream topped with coffee and raisin sauce.

Snack 1 ☐ *1 small slice wholemeal bread, 25g/1oz* *50g/2oz liver pâté* *1 tomato*

Toast bread and spread with liver pâté. Top with tomato.

Snack 2 ☐ *150ml/¼ pint whole milk or 275ml/½ pint skimmed milk* *2 large digestive biscuits*

☐ If you completed the day without cheating at all, tick here and move on to Day 20.

☐ If you cheated, do a 'Saintly Day' tomorrow (page 253) instead of the set menu.

☐ If you do not eat one meal or snack that you are allowed, tick this box and save up for a 'Naughty Day'. When you have two ticks saved, you can do any of the Thoroughly Naughty Day's Menus *instead* of your next day's diet.

Exercise Day 19

MORNING ☐ Repeat Exercise 1: 5 times

☐ Repeat Exercise 2: 5 times to right
5 times to left

☐ Repeat Exercise 3: 5 times circling left and right with right foot
☐ 5 times circling left and right with left foot

☐ Repeat Exercise 4: touch the floor 15 times

☐ Repeat Exercise 5: bend to the left and right 15 times

☐ Repeat Exercise 6: circle to left 15 times
circle to right 15 times

☐ Repeat Exercise 7: criss-cross 20 times

☐ Repeat Exercise 8: stretch 5 times

☐ Repeat Exercise 9: touch left foot and sit up
touch right foot and sit up 15 times

☐ Repeat Exercise 10: floor-walk to wall and back twice

LUNCHTIME ☐ Walk for 23 minutes marking your position 3 minutes from starting point. Turn and briskly walk to your marked place in 16 minutes then jog the final stretch.

EVENING ☐ Run to the top of the stairs and down again 4 times. Jog for 10 minutes.
If you are jogging on the spot or around the house, lift your legs and knees up as high as you can manage. This is much more strenuous than if you barely lift your feet from the floor.

Or ☐ Jog for 19 minutes:
1st 5-minute jog
2nd 5-minute jog
3rd 5-minute jog
4th 4-minute jog

Then ☐ Skip 75 times.

Bedtime Relaxer ☐

Beauty Day 19

Eye care
Eyes are mostly strong and healthy and work efficiently without any extra help. Although actual sight is unaffected

by late nights, tiredness or a smoky atmosphere can leave eyes red and dark-ringed.

Faces have some natural built-in protection against overhead glare. Brows, browbone and eyelids act as a kind of visor. But eyes have no defence against low-level glare, from strong light bouncing off sand, sea and the white concrete structures of towns and cities, so sunlight can affect them. They need protection from more penetrating rays, such as ultra violet and infra red. These are present in all sunlight and especially in the potent light of tropical climes, and can be overcome by wearing dark lenses. The sunshine of a British summer is usually less fierce and sunglasses with lighter lenses help prevent discomfort while ensuring clear vision. An urge to squint is the signal that eyes *need* protection from sunlight. They may begin to ache as muscles which usually work spasmodically — controlling blink rate, for example — are kept in a constant state of tension. Choice of the colour of lenses is less important than lack of distortion. A simple test can reveal flaws in non-prescription lenses. Hold frames at arm's length. Concentrate on one lens at a time and focus on a straight, upright object ahead. Rotate the glasses slowly. If your 'marker' appears distorted, the lens is flawed. Reject those glasses.

Looking fresh and bright-eyed is mostly a matter of making yourself comfortable. It's much less tiring to read with the light behind you than to have it shining in your eyes. It's also easier to keep a low-wattage light on when watching television to offset the glare. If your eyes feel tired during a long bout of close work, raise your head and focus on some long-distance object. Then look up, look right, downwards, left and up again. Repeat this 3 or 4 times. For a quick refresher, increase your blink rate.

Eyes have a built-in sprinkler system, the lachrymal gland, which produces tears to wash away irritants. So eye baths are mostly unnecessary. There are times, however, when eyes may need extra help; perhaps when the disinfectant in swimming baths or the dust from roads leave them sore. A mild saline soother can be made as follows: mix a teaspoon of fine kitchen salt with a pint of water and boil for 3 minutes. Cover and leave to cool. Use it as you would any eye bath, tepidly warm.

Today's special treatment
A cool toner for tired eyes. Try it now and repeat the treatment whenever your eyes need a wide-awake look.

Make up the saline solution above, and leave in the refrigerator for 20 minutes. Dip 2 large pads of cotton wool into the saline and squeeze out any surplus. Lie down with the pads over your eyes for 10 minutes.

Frames to flatter faces

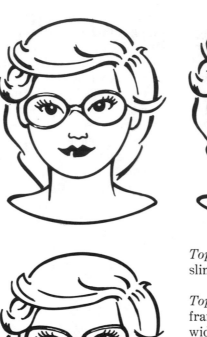
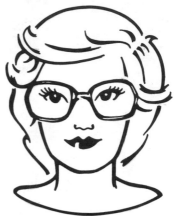

Top Left For a round face: slim oval frames.

Top Right For a long face: frames with depth and width.

Left For a square face: softly-rounded frames, slightly upswept.

Cleanse, tone moisturize ☐	Cleanse, tone and moisturize your face in the morning and at night.
Hair livener ☐	For dry hair only: massage scalp, see page 61, Day 7, but omit oil.
Spotty back? ☐	Soak in warm bath; scrub back with medicated soap, dry and dab with diluted antiseptic. Dust with medicated talc.

Shopping Checklist Day 20

Choose your meals, then write in by each relevant item the amount you require.

Amount required	*Amount required*	*Amount required*
Fruit and Vegetables	Eggs	Mustard
Baby beets	Low-fat natural	Oil
Carrots	yogurt	Oil-free French
Cucumber	Low-fat spread	dressing
Green beans	Parmesan cheese	Salt and pepper
Onion	Skimmed milk	Stock cube
Peas	**Grocery**	Sugar
Tomatoes	Baked beans in	Sweet pickle
Watercress	tomato sauce	
Banana	Bran breakfast cereal	
Blackberries	Crisps	
Cooking apple	Currant bun	
Orange	Digestive biscuit	
Plums	Dried apricots	
Frozen Foods	French bread	
Green beans	Macaroni	
Peas	Pasta shells	
Meat, Poultry and Fish	Prunes	
Calves' or lamb's	Rice	
liver	Spaghetti in tomato	
Streaky bacon	sauce	
Dairy Produce/Eggs	Tuna canned in brine	
Cheddar, Cheshire or	Wholemeal bread	
Wensleydale cheese	**Store Cupboard**	
Edam or Tendale	Cornflour	
cheese	Marmalade	

Diet Day 20

☐ *275ml/½ pint skimmed milk or reconstituted low-fat powdered milk*

BREAKFAST/SUPPER MEAL

Either ☐ *2 eggs, size 3; 25ml/1 tablespoon skimmed milk (extra to allowance); 1 tomato*
Scramble eggs in a non-stick pan with milk. Serve with tomato grilled without fat.

Or ☐ *25g/1oz any bran breakfast cereal; 60ml/4 tablespoons low-fat natural yogurt; 2 dried apricots, chopped*

Or ☐ *1 small slice wholemeal bread, 25g/1oz, toasted; 150g/5.3oz can baked beans in tomato sauce*
Heat beans and serve on toast.

LIGHT MEAL

Either to eat at home **Spaghetti and Cheese plus Fruit and Yogurt**
☐ *213g/7½oz can spaghetti in tomato sauce*
15ml/1 level tablespoon grated Parmesan cheese
1 small carton low-fat natural yogurt
2 dessert plums or 3 prunes
Heat spaghetti and serve sprinkled with Parmesan cheese. Follow with yogurt mixed with fruit.

Or to take to work **Tuna and Pasta Salad plus Biscuits**
☐ *25g/1oz pasta shells, raw*
2 baby beets
¼ cucumber
15ml/1 tablespoon oil-free French dressing
100g/3½oz tuna canned in brine
1 digestive biscuit
Boil pasta shells until cooked, then drain. Rinse in cold water and drain again. Mix pasta with diced beets and cucumber and dressing. Drain tuna, flake and add to pasta mixture. Take to work in a plastic container. Follow with biscuit.

Or if you prefer to eat vegetarian **Cheese and Pickle Sandwich plus Carrot Sticks**
☐ *50g/2oz French bread or 2 small slices wholemeal bread, 25g/1oz each*
15ml/1 level tablespoon sweet pickle
25g/1oz Cheddar, Cheshire or Wensleydale cheese
50g/2oz carrots

161

Spread bread with pickle and make into a sandwich with cheese. Eat with raw carrots cut into sticks.

MAIN MEAL

Either a quick meal
Grilled Liver and Bacon plus Fruit

75g/3oz calves' or lamb's liver
1 rasher streaky bacon
2 tomatoes
115g/4oz peas, fresh or frozen

Watercress (optional)
1 small cooking apple
50g/2oz blackberries
10ml/2 level teaspoons sugar

Thinly slice liver and grill with bacon and tomatoes without adding any fat. Boil peas and serve with liver, bacon, tomatoes and watercress. Peel, core and slice the apple. Stew with blackberries, sugar and a little water.

Or a keen cook's recipe
Liver with Orange and Rice

75g/3oz calves' or lamb's liver
25g/1oz rice, raw
115g/4oz green beans, sliced, fresh or frozen
5ml/1 teaspoon oil
½ small onion

5ml/1 level teaspoon cornflour
Salt and pepper
Pinch dry mustard
150ml/¼ pint stock made with stock cube
1 medium orange

Thinly slice liver. Boil the rice and green beans. Heat oil in a non-stick pan and add the liver and chopped onion. Cook gently for about 10 minutes, turning liver to brown each side. Remove liver and keep hot. Add cornflour, seasoning and mustard to the pan and, stirring, add the stock. Bring to the boil and simmer for 1 minute. Pour over the liver. Serve with rice and green beans and half the orange cut into segments. Eat the second orange half for dessert.

Or if you prefer to eat vegetarian
Macaroni Cheese

50g/2oz macaroni
150ml/¼ pint skimmed milk
10ml/2 level teaspoons cornflour
10ml/2 level teaspoons low-fat spread

Pinch dry mustard
Salt and pepper
25g/1oz Edam or Tendale cheese
1 tomato

Cook the macaroni in boiling salted water until tender, then drain. Put the milk, cornflour and low-fat spread into a small saucepan and heat, whisking all the time until the sauce thickens. Season to taste with salt and pepper. Stir in the mustard and grated cheese. Mix with the cooked macaroni and turn into a small heatproof dish. Top with slices of tomato and brown under a hot grill.

Snack 1 ☐ *1 small packet crisps, any*   *25g/1oz Cheddar cheese*
flavour

Snack 2 ☐ *1 currant bun, 50g/1¾oz*   *1 small banana*
10ml/2 level teaspoons low-
fat spread

☐ If you completed the day without cheating at all, tick here and move on to Day 21.

☐ If you cheated, do a 'Saintly Day' tomorrow (page 253) instead of the set menu.

☐ If you do not eat one meal or snack that you are allowed, tick this box and save up for a 'Naughty Day'. When you have two ticks saved, you can do any of the Thoroughly Naughty Day's Menus *instead* of your next day's diet.

Exercise Day 20

MORNING ☐ Repeat Exercise 1: 5 times

☐ Repeat Exercise 2: 5 times to right
5 times to left

☐ Repeat Exercise 3: 5 times circling left and right with right foot
5 times circling left and right with left foot

☐ Repeat Exercise 4: touch the floor 15 times

☐ Repeat Exercise 5: bend to left and right 15 times

☐ Repeat Exercise 6: circle to left 15 times
circle to right 15 times

☐ Repeat Exercise 7: criss-cross 20 times

☐ Repeat Exercise 8: stretch 5 times

☐ Repeat Exercise 9: touch left foot and sit up
touch right foot and sit up 15 times

☐ Repeat Exercise 10: floor-walk to wall and back 3 times
*Lift your left then right buttock off the floor as you move
backwards and forwards. If you put lots of effort into this
exercise it's a great calorie burner.*

LUNCHTIME ☐ Walk for 24 minutes, marking your position 4 minutes from
your starting point. Turn and briskly walk to your marked
place in 16 minutes then jog the final stretch.

EVENING ☐ Run to top of stairs and down again 4 times. Jog for 10
minutes.

Or ☐ Jog for 20 minutes:
1st 5-minute jog
2nd 5-minute jog
3rd 5-minute jog
4th 5-minute jog

Then ☐ Skip 100 times.

Bedtime Relaxer ☐

Beauty Day 20

Artful make-up can transform your eyes, so it's worth
taking time to discover how to give them the right kind of
emphasis.

Eye pencils
The latest pencils are soft-centred for using on the delicate
skin round eyes, and come in many shades. Look for dark
muted brown, which flatters most eye colouring and is a
good choice for shaping. Avoid a reddish brown.

Eyeshadows
These are available in cream, liquid or powder form.
Powder block colour is one of the easiest to use. Many
include their own applicator but you may find that you can
achieve a softer look by using a size-3 paintbrush to blend

the colour. Cosmetic brushes, available from chemists, come
in a similar size.

Eyeliners
Eyeliner should be used sparingly. A heavy line round eyes
makes them appear smaller and it can be hard and ageing.
Keep eyeliner mainly to outer corners, tracing a fine line
close to lash roots. Many models prefer to use cake eyeliner.
This should be moistened and then applied with a finely-
tipped brush. The trick is to keep your hand steady — it
helps if you rest your elbow on a firm surface.

Mascaras
These are mostly sold in slim cylinders. Some contain tiny
brushes but those with a rod are easier to handle and can be
used to thicken and curl lashes.

Reshaping eyes

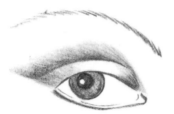 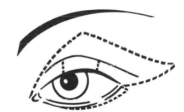

A. *For small eyes* Shade along socket line, beginning a little way in from inner
eye. Brush colour upwards and outwards. Stroke a very
pale colour along upper lids and blend into socket shading.
Shade finely under outer lid. Highlight centre of upper lid
with pale or pearly colour.

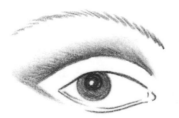 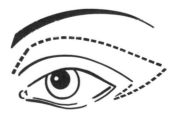

B. *Deep-set eyes* Highlight upper lid generously. Blend a deeper but neutral
sludgy shade from socket line upwards to fade near brow.

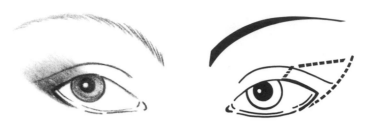

C. *Close-set eyes* Widen them with eyeliner at outer corners and shading drawn outwards.

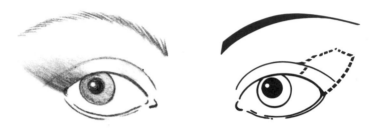

D. *Round eyes* Shade strongly at outer corners. Blend up and outwards.

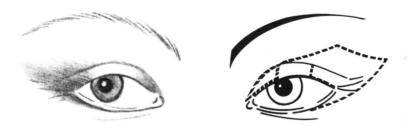

E. *Not-so-young eyes, droopy lids* Shade upwards at outer corners. Highlight softly at centre of lids.

Today's special treatment
Experiment with your eye make-up until you find what suits you best. Do not be afraid to mix eye colours, but make sure you blend them together where they meet. If you don't normally wear eye make-up, start off your collection with tones of brown and grey. They'll shade your eyes very naturally and suit any colour content. It's not always necessary to match eye colour to the clothes you wear, a contrast often works well. Turquoise shadow with a

beige outfit, for example. Or brown eye shadow with a red outfit. Here are a few extra tips on applying eye make-up.

1. Apply eye colour from centre of lid, pencilling or painting outwards.

2. Soften the colour outwards and upwards with a clean brush.

3. Apply colour under lower lashes and smudge with a brush to soften.

4. Glance downwards. Brush mascara down from roots to tips on top of upper lashes. Brush from under and up. Brush lower lids downwards.

Cleanse, tone, moisturize

Cleanse, tone and moisturize your face in the morning and at night.

Hair livener

Massage scalp, see page 61, Day 7, but omit oil.

Neck treat

Repeat treatment on page 49, Day 5.

Shopping Checklist Day 21

Choose your meals, then write in by each relevant item the amount you require.

Amount required	*Amount required*	*Amount required*
Fruit and Vegetables	**Dairy Produce/Eggs**	Stock cube
Carrots	Cheese spread	Tomato purée
Green pepper	Curd cheese	
Mushrooms	Eggs	
Onion	Low-fat fruit yogurt	
Peas	Low-fat natural	
Potato	yogurt	
Swede	Low-fat spread	
Tomatoes	Skimmed milk	
Apple	**Grocery**	
Banana	Bran breakfast cereal	
Grapefruit	Crispbreads	
Grapes	Cucumber or	
Orange	onion relish	
Pear	Digestive biscuit	
Frozen Foods	Instant potato powder	
Sliced roast beef	Sweet pickle	
in gravy	Wholemeal bread	
Mixed vegetables	Yeast extract	
Peas	**Store Cupboard**	
Meat, Poultry and Fish	Cornflour	
Chipolata sausages	Jam	
Corned beef	Low-calorie salad	
Roast beef	dressing	
Stewing beef	Mixed herbs	
Streaky bacon	Salt and pepper	

Diet Day 21

☐ *275ml/½ pint skimmed milk or reconstituted low-fat powdered milk*

BREAKFAST/SUPPER MEAL

Either ☐ *1 small slice wholemeal bread, 25g/1oz; 1 egg, size 3; 5ml/1 level teaspoon low-fat spread*
Dip bread into beaten egg and fry in a non-stick pan greased with low-fat spread.

Or ☐ *25g/1oz any bran breakfast cereal; 75ml/5 tablespoons skimmed milk (extra to allowance); 1 small orange*

Or ☐ *2 tomatoes, well grilled without fat; 2 rashers streaky bacon, well grilled; 1 small slice wholemeal bread, 25g/1oz*

LIGHT MEAL

Either to eat at home **Hot Dogs plus Apple** ☐

2 beef or pork chipolata sausages	*15ml/1 level tablespoon cucumber or onion relish*
2 small slices wholemeal bread, 25g/1oz each	*1 medium apple*

Grill sausages well. Spread slices of bread with relish and roll up one sausage in each slice. Follow with apple.

Or to take to work **Corned Beef and Pickle Sandwich plus Pear** ☐

2 small slices wholemeal bread, 25g/1oz each	*40g/1½oz corned beef*
15ml/1 tablespoon sweet pickle	*2 tomatoes*
	1 pear

Spread bread with pickle and make a sandwich with corned beef. Eat sandwich with tomatoes and follow with pear.

Or if you prefer to eat vegetarian **Vegetable Salad with Cheese Crispbread** ☐

175g/6oz mixed vegetables, frozen	*30ml/2 tablespoons low-fat natural yogurt*
30ml/2 tablespoons low-calorie salad dressing	*25g/1oz cheese spread*
	2 crispbreads

Boil mixed vegetables for 5 minutes, then drain and rinse under cold water. Drain again and put into a container. Mix salad dressing with yogurt and add to vegetables. Eat salad with crispbreads and cheese spread.

*Either a
quick recipe*
**Roast Beef
with Vegetables
plus Grapes**

*100g/3½oz lean roast beef or
    113g/4oz packet frozen
    sliced roast beef in gravy
50g/2oz peas, boiled
75g/3oz carrots, boiled*

*150g/5oz potato, boiled
115g/4oz grapes
15ml/1 level tablespoon low-
    fat natural yogurt*

Serve beef with vegetables. Cut grapes in half and top with yogurt.

---

*Or a keen
cook's recipe*
**Beef Stew
plus Cheese
Surprise**

*75g/3oz very lean stewing
    beef
50g/2oz mushrooms
1 small onion
50g/2oz swede
50g/2oz carrot
Salt and pepper
Pinch mixed herbs
10ml/2 level teaspoons
    tomato purée*

*5ml/1 level teaspoon
    cornflour
150ml/¼ pint stock made
    with stock cube
30ml/2 level tablespoons
    instant potato powder
1 digestive biscuit
5ml/1 level teaspoon jam
15g/½oz curd cheese*

Cube beef and slice mushrooms and onion. Dice swede and carrot. Put meat and vegetables in a casserole dish with tomato purée and herbs. Mix cornflour with stock and add to casserole. Season. Cover dish and cook at 300°F/150°C, gas mark 3, for 2 hours. Make up the potato powder with water and serve with beef stew. To follow, spread biscuit with jam and top with curd cheese.

---

*Or if you
prefer to eat
vegetarian*
**Piperade plus
Banana**

*1 tomato
2 eggs, size 3
30ml/2 level tablespoons
    skimmed milk
Salt and pepper
15ml/1 level tablespoon low-
    fat spread*

*½ green pepper
2 small slices wholemeal
    bread, 25g/1oz each
1 small banana*

Stand tomato in boiling water for a few minutes, then remove skin. Chop flesh. Beat eggs with skimmed milk and season. Pour mixture into a non-stick pan with low-fat spread and stir until scrambled. Just before eggs are fully cooked, stir in tomato and sliced green pepper. Stir until eggs are cooked. Serve on toasted bread. Follow with banana.

Snack 1

*1 small orange
1 medium grapefruit*

*1 low-fat fruit yogurt,
    any flavour*

Either eat separately or make the following cocktail. Cut

grapefruit in half, remove flesh and cut into cubes. Peel and segment orange and add to grapefruit. Mix with yogurt and spoon back into grapefruit halves.

Snack 2 ☐ *4 crispbreads*   *65g/2½oz curd cheese*
           20ml/4 level teaspoons yeast   *2 tomatoes*
             extract
Spread crispbreads with yeast extract and top with curd cheese. Eat with tomatoes.

☐ If you completed the day without cheating at all, tick here and move on to Day 22.

☐ If you cheated, do a 'Saintly Day' tomorrow (page 253) instead of the set menu.

☐ If you do not eat one meal or snack that you are allowed, tick this box and save up for a 'Naughty Day'. When you have two ticks saved, you can do any of the Thoroughly Naughty Day's Menus *instead* of your next day's diet.

Exercise Day 21

MORNING ☐ Repeat Exercise 1: 5 times

☐ Repeat Exercise 2: 5 times to right
   5 times to left

☐ Repeat Exercise 3: 5 times circling left and right with right foot
   5 times circling left and right with left foot

☐ Repeat Exercise 4: touch the floor 15 times

☐ Repeat Exercise 5: bend to left and right 15 times

☐ Repeat Exercise 6: circle to left 15 times
   circle to right 15 times

171

☐ Repeat Exercise 7: criss-cross 20 times

☐ Repeat Exercise 8: stretch 5 times

☐ Repeat Exercise 9: touch left foot and sit up
touch right foot and sit up 15 times

☐ Repeat Exercise 10: floor-walk to wall and back 4 times

LUNCHTIME ☐ Walk for 25 minutes marking your position 5 minutes from your starting point. Turn and briskly walk to your marked place in 16 minutes then jog the final stretch.

EVENING ☐ Run to top of stairs and down again 4 times. Jog for 10 minutes.

Or ☐ Jog for 20 minutes:
1st 5-minute jog
2nd 5-minute jog
3rd 5-minute jog
4th 5-minute jog

Then ☐ Skip 125 times.
If you keep tripping over your skipping rope, it could be the wrong length for you. Experiment with it longer or shorter and see if this improves your performance.

Bedtime Relaxer ☐

Beauty Day 21

There's nothing more welcoming than a smile. It's reassuring, puts others at their ease, and a confident smile makes any face instantly more attractive. But you won't smile easily if you have doubts about your teeth. Discount those stories about people who neglect their teeth and never suffer a twinge. Some teeth *are* stronger and seemingly more able to resist decay than others; but ply any teeth with sugary foods and ignore dental hygiene, and your smile will suffer. Problems start with sticky plaque. Left undetected, plaque builds up in the mouth and converts sugar into acids which attack tooth enamel. You can see how plaque clings by using a dental disclosing product sold by chemists. This tints the plaque, and shows how it sites itself near gums which can eventually become infected and loosen teeth. But this need never happen. Proper cleaning and regular 6-monthly visits to the dentist can ensure that any danger is dealt with.

Brush for shine
Thoroughly brush your teeth at night and in the morning. Also brush your teeth after you have eaten. Ask your dentist to recommend the best toothbrush for your teeth. A soft toothbrush with fine filaments will reach the parts that rigid brushes can't.

Embarrassed by your teeth?
Well, they don't have to be perfect to produce a warm smile. They may be larger or less evenly spaced than those you see in the toothpaste advertisements, but then most teeth are.

If your teeth are discoloured or misshapen, you should talk this over with your dentist. An ugly tooth can be fined down and 'capped' by a natural-looking crown and no one need know that it isn't a natural tooth. This is referred to as cosmetic dentistry, and is rarely available on the National Health Service. As you may have to pay a sizeable private fee, there is no reason why you should not consult more than one dentist and compare estimates.

Lip colour
Bright colour draws attention to your mouth, so if you have anything to hide, pick a soft, but not pale, shade. The brighter colours look luscious on young, rounded lips but on a thinner, down-turning mouth they can be too severe. Creamy textured lipstick is kinder than frosted lip colour which tends to emphasize little lines. Soft coral pinks are gentle and flattering.

Today's special treatment
Identify with one of the mouth shapes on the next page and practise improving your mouth.

A. *This way for a pretty mouth*

Shape upper lip by outlining from centre to outer corners. Outline lower lip from corner to corner. Fill in the outline with lip colour, using your lipstick or painting with a lip brush. The experts use a lip brush to achieve a precise outline, but you may find it easier to do this with a lip pencil. Lip pencils are available in several shades and your outline should be in a slightly darker colour than the inside colour. For correcting lip shape: a beige brown.

B. *Lips too thick?*

Outline with brownish pencil just inside the natural lip shape. Colour in with lipstick.

C. *Lips too thin?*

You can make lips plumper with stronger colour. Outline fractionally outside the natural lip line. If you use a lip pencil, choose red. Colour in with toning lipstick. For a more subtle effect, blot after colouring by placing a tissue between lips and pressing lips together. Paint on a softer colour up to lip line.

D. *Drooping mouth?*

Make lower lip fuller by lining with brownish pencil outside natural contour. Lift colour slightly at upper lip corners. Colour in with lipstick.

E. *Wrinkled lips?* ☐ Stretch lips with finger and thumb, then outline with a skin-toned pencil to help prevent lip colour smudging into lines outside mouth. Release lips and colour in with lipstick.

Cleanse, tone, moisturize ☐ Cleanse, tone and moisturize your face in the morning and at night.

Hair livener ☐ For dry hair only: massage scalp, see page 61, Day 7, but omit oil.

Elbows ☐ Still rough or discoloured? Mix lemon juice with a little salt and rub in. Rinse off after 5 to 10 minutes and apply body lotion.

Spotty back? ☐ Soak in warm bath; scrub back with medicated soap, dry and dab with diluted antiseptic. Dust with medicated talc.

Manicure ☐ Repeat manicure from page 54, Day 6.

How to get what you want

If a woman is well informed about dieting techniques yet
remains defeated by a weight problem she cannot control,
however much she might say that she wants to conquer it,
there is usually something in the long-term goal that
disturbs her. The way to find out is to ask the question:
'What are you gaining from staying overweight?' Most
women are horrified by this. 'How can you ask such a thing?'
they exclaim. 'Why, being overweight is ruining my life!'
But when we probe a little deeper into those hidden
feelings, we find that there are usually factors involved
which the subconscious mind construes as benefits. When a
woman starts to lose a lot of weight, other people are going
to change their attitudes towards her. They have to do
some adjusting to this new person, this butterfly emerging
from the chrysalis. Some will be a bit disturbed or uneasy,
some will be critical. Others will give whole-hearted
approval. What nobody will do is ignore it! Many women
who diet successfully thrive on the extra attention. They
see it, quite rightly, as due interest in the more exciting and
confident person they have become. But others may find it
disturbing. While they stay fat, life is predictable, with no
challenges to upset the status quo. They might not enjoy
being overweight, but it is 'safe'.

Of course, not every woman needs or wants to lose a
great deal of weight. But most of us do want ourselves or
our lives to alter in some way that makes us more fulfilled
and complete, and thus happier. We have never met anybody who couldn't name at least 3 things she (or he) would
like to change. Improved health . . . a more interesting life
. . . more fun . . . more scope . . . more people . . . wider
interests. They are the things we all need in order to thrive
and flourish.

A restless feeling is usually very healthy. There is
nothing wrong and everything right with a desire to give
more to life and get more out of it. If you have this feeling,
the next question to ask yourself is: 'What is it in my
present environment that is not totally satisfying? Why am
I feeling restless? What is missing in my day-to-day
existence?' Once you have the answers you are already
more than halfway to knowing how to make a change for
the better. But will you do it? It's tempting to believe that if
only a fairy godmother would come along and wave a wand
and confer heaps of gold, a fantastic job, a fine new home,

etc., everything would be 'different'. But it wouldn't. The
only worthwhile changes we can ever make to improve our
lives and give us more fulfilment are the ones we make in
ourselves. They don't depend on circumstances, and they
don't depend on other people.

Your first step to happiness is to recognize this truth:
that if you are overweight, or in the wrong job, or
frustrated in doing some of the things you would like to do,
it truly isn't anybody else's fault. Not ever. Your happiness
and your fulfilment are your responsibility.

Many women say that they can't possibly keep to a diet
because they have to provide a good table for the family.
But it isn't the family that forces all those extra calories
down your throat. Some women believe that while life is
extra difficult — their husbands out of work, for instance,
or the children going through a bad time at school — there
is no point trying to improve anything. Because most
women feel responsible for the happiness of those close to
them, this attitude is very understandable. But it doesn't
help. However hard your circumstances, you must keep a
corner of life for yourself and your own growth as a human
being. If you let yourself get swamped by the needs of
others, there is less of you to give. And, sooner or later, you
find yourself on the spiral slope down to depression. We all
need to grow, we all need to discover and develop those
parts of our nature that nourish us, and if you simply sit
back and let life happen to you, you just become one of life's
victims.

What is it, then, that so often inhibits us from taking
steps to make our lives more fulfilling? Curiously, it has
something to do with the nature of change itself. Change
equals challenge. It is a challenge to disturb the
'comfortable' pattern of things as they are. A challenge that
calls on each of us, and nobody else, to put our wits and
willpower to the test so as to improve our lives. Many
people draw back from a challenge, even when it is a
comparatively easy one like enrolling in an evening class or
a slimming club, and there are good reasons for this. The
first one is to be found in our own human nature. It is an
interesting fact, well known to psychiatrists, that we tend
to react quite powerfully to any factors that look as if they
might disturb the pattern of our lives. It is easier, as a rule,
to hold on fast to our habits and our day-to-day routine than
to let go and make new things happen.

In fact, so strongly do we react to changes (whether
forced on us or made by ourselves), that alterations in
lifestyle, status or habits constitute some of the major

stresses of life. You may be surprised to learn that even happy events like getting married or promotion at work provide a stress reaction: so do such other potential improvements as giving up smoking or embarking on a diet.

But what is stress? Most people think of it in terms of knotted brows and sleepless nights — but it doesn't always necessarily have an adverse effect. Stress is also another word for stimulation: an invigorating shot of adrenalin that helps us accept the new demands on our energy and get on with life. Some people thrive on the stress that challenges bring. Others don't. Some women actively fear all challenges and changes, and this brings us to the second reason why it can be difficult to embark on a new venture. We all tend to fill the unknown with our own personal predictions. Women who are afraid of changing anything, even when they secretly long to, have very little faith in themselves. Deep down, they don't think much of their claims on life, often because of unhappy past experiences. Perhaps they were made to feel inadequate or a nuisance to others when they were children and continue to carry a negative self-image into adult life, too. They project these inner feelings of uncertainty and failure into the future.

Even if, in the past, you have had bad 'luck' in your relationships, in your job or with your weight-loss plan, there's no reason why you should fail in the future. Look at your life as it is today, and you'll see that the future always holds more promise than the past — if you can bring yourself to seize the opportunities now.

However hard you try to protect yourself, and to keep everything as it is, it simply can't be done. Life doesn't stand still. Each day you wake up, you are a day older — and what that day holds is largely up to you. People don't ever stay where you want them, or even the way you want them to be. What you do with your life is for you to choose. The temptation to cling on, to put up with life as it is rather than risk the effort to grow in your own right, should be resisted — because if you give in to it, the only person who suffers in the end is you. But if you do take up the challenge of changing, the rewards are greater than you may imagine.

Your 7-point chart for change

1. First, establish your aims. Take pen and paper now and write down the changes you want. Not the changes you think you ought to make to please somebody else, but those you desire for yourself. This is a wonderful way of clearing out the cobwebs and getting things straight.

2. Face up to any attached risks. You'll find out what they are if you now write down all the pros and cons for making each change. If there are more items in the con column, you'll probably decide not to go ahead with a particular change — but at least you'll know why! If you do decide to go ahead, now you can start planning.

3. Write down the point you are at. That's Point A. Now write down the goal you aim for. That's Point B. Suppose you are 2st overweight, and should weigh 9st. Point A is then '11st'. Point B is '9st'. Suppose you have always wanted to speak good French. Point A might be 'schoolgirl French at present'. Point B would be 'to speak French fluently'.

4. Whatever your goal, how are you going to get there? Go through from Point A to Point B in slow motion. Work out all the steps you need to take; and you will see that the only thing you have to do now is take the first step.

This is a vital exercise because it helps you be realistic. It's lack of realism that spoils so many good plans and is the biggest stumbling block to success in any undertaking, however large or small.

5. Do expect other people to react to the change in you — not always with unqualified approval, either! It is another curious fact about our resistance to change that we don't always feel comfortable when we see it in others. We like (or don't like) others, and they fit into our perspective because they are what they are; in all our relationships, we have found a balance that depends on the other person staying the same. If that other person starts to change — to become more assertive, for instance, or to look different — it can throw us. We have to adjust to this new human being who no longer fits our old image of him or her. Quite often, people instinctively try to encourage this 'new' person to revert to their former self, so that their relationship can follow its old, familiar pattern.

If you do decide to change your shape or your ways you must expect some people to offer criticism, but others will undoubtedly love and applaud you for the alteration.

6. Don't expect rewards immediately. The change you are making may seem cataclysmic and world-shaking to you, but it's most unlikely to bring you instant success and confidence, or instant happiness . . . any more than a diet, however strict, is going to result in the instant loss of all

that surplus weight. Compare it to climbing a ladder —
from every rung the view changes, and even at the halfway stage you can look down and back at where you were
and congratulate yourself.

7. Be prepared for difficulties. If you are trying to change
your habits, it won't always come easy. Nobody likes
obstacles, and sloth is just as popular today as it ever was.
But there is never going to be a time when a change for the
better will just happen without effort. Still, make it as easy
for yourself as you can . . . and do try not to let the slips or
problems of today spoil your attempts to create a better
future. It's there waiting for you.

Week 4

☐☐	Weigh yourself and write in your weight here
☐☐	Now check the chart on page 7 and write in your ideal weight here
☐☐	Write in the amount you have to lose here

Now tick one of these boxes, and this is your menu plan for this week

☐ If you have under 1st to lose, you can have breakfast/supper, a light meal and a main meal each day.

☐ If you have between 1st and 3st to lose, you can have breakfast/supper, a light meal, a main meal and one snack.

☐ If you have over 3st to lose, you can have breakfast/supper, a light meal, a main meal and two snacks.

Shopping Checklist Day 22

Choose your meals, then write in by each relevant item the amount you require.

Amount required	Amount required	Amount required
Fruit and Vegetables	Eggs	Vinegar
Cabbage	Low-fat natural	
Carrot	yogurt	
Celery	Low-fat spread	
Chicory	Skimmed milk	
Lettuce	**Grocery**	
Mushrooms	Bran breakfast cereal	
Onion	Corn snacks	
Peas	Muesli or fruit	
Potato	and nut bar	
Tomatoes	Onion or corn relish	
Watercress	Raisins or sultanas	
Banana	Ravioli in beef	
Orange	and tomato sauce	
Peach	Wholemeal bread	
Frozen Foods	Wholemeal roll	
Peas	**Store Cupboard**	
Water ice or sorbet	Cornflour	
Meat, Poultry and Fish	Horseradish sauce	
Chicken breast	Low-calorie salad	
Chipolata sausages	dressing	
Kidneys	Salt and pepper	
Dairy Produce/Eggs	Stock cube	
Curd cheese	Sweet pickle	
Edam or Tendale	Tomato ketchup	
cheese	Tomato purée	

Diet Day 22

☐ *275ml/½ pint skimmed milk or reconstituted low-fat powdered milk*

Either ☐ *2 tomatoes, grilled without fat; 2 beef or pork chipolata sausages, well grilled; 1 small slice wholemeal bread, 25g/1oz*

Or ☐ *1 egg, size 3, boiled; 1 small slice wholemeal bread, 25g/1oz; 5ml/1 level teaspoon low-fat spread*

Or ☐ *25g/1oz any bran breakfast cereal; 75ml/5 tablespoons skimmed milk (extra to allowance); 30ml/2 level tablespoons raisins or sultanas*

LIGHT MEAL

Either to eat at home
Ravioli and Cheese plus Fruit

☐ *215g/7.6oz can ravioli in beef and tomato sauce* *15ml/1 level tablespoon fresh wholemeal breadcrumbs*
25g/1oz Edam or Tendale cheese *1 small orange or peach*

Heat ravioli and place in an ovenproof dish. Grate cheese and mix with breadcrumbs. Sprinkle on top of ravioli and grill. Follow with fruit.

Or to take to work
Egg and Cheese Roll plus Fruit

☐ *1 egg, size 3* *1 stick celery*
15ml/1 tablespoon low-calorie salad dressing *2 tomatoes*
Watercress
Salt and pepper *Chicory or lettuce*
25g/1oz curd cheese *1 small orange or peach*
1 wholemeal roll, 50g/2oz

Hard boil the egg; cool under cold water tap; shell and mash with salad dressing. Season to taste. Spread curd cheese on roll and fill with egg mixture. Chop celery and tomatoes and mix with a few sprigs of watercress and sliced chicory or lettuce leaves. Take salad to work in separate container and eat with roll. Follow with fruit.

Either an easy recipe **Kidney-stuffed Potato plus Water Ice**

200g/7oz potato
2 lambs' kidneys
Stock made from stock cube
75g/3oz red or white cabbage
Salt and pepper

15ml/1 level tablespoon sweet pickle .
50g/2oz water ice or sorbet, any flavour

Scrub potato and bake in its jacket at 200°C/400°F, gas mark 6, for 40 minutes, or until soft when pinched. Halve and core the kidneys and poach them in a little stock until cooked. Chop cabbage and boil in salted water until cooked. Halve potato and scoop out flesh into a bowl. Chop kidneys and add to potato. Season and pile back into potato shells. Serve with boiled cabbage and pickle. Follow with water ice or sorbet.

Or a keen cook's recipe **Mushroom Cocktail and Chicken Casserole**

15ml/1 tablespoon tomato ketchup
5ml/1 teaspoon vinegar
2.5ml/½ level teaspoon horseradish sauce
Lettuce
115g/4oz mushrooms
75g/3oz boned chicken breast
1 small onion
150ml/¼ pint stock made with stock cube

5ml/1 level teaspoon cornflour
10ml/2 teaspoons tomato purée
150g/5oz potato
30ml/2 tablespoons skimmed milk
115g/4oz peas, fresh or frozen

Mix tomato ketchup with vinegar and horseradish sauce. Line a glass dish with shredded lettuce. Slice four small mushrooms and place on top of lettuce. Cover with ketchup mixture and chill. Start your meal with the mushroom cocktail. Remove skin from chicken and cut meat into cubes. Put in a saucepan with the remaining mushrooms cut into slices and chopped onion. Add stock and bring to the boil. Add tomato purée and simmer for about 45 minutes. Mix cornflour with a little cold water and add to chicken. Boil until thickened. Boil potato and mash with skimmed milk. Boil peas and serve with chicken and potatoes.

Or if you prefer to eat vegetarian **Mushroom-stuffed Potato with Coleslaw**

200g/7oz potato
50g/2oz mushrooms
15ml/1 level tablespoon onion or corn relish
115g/4oz white cabbage
1 carrot

15ml/1 tablespoon low-calorie salad dressing
30ml/2 level tablespoons low-fat natural yogurt
1 medium banana

Scrub potato and bake in its jacket at 200°C/400°F, gas mark 6, for 40 minutes or until soft when pinched. Thinly slice mushrooms. Cut potato in half lengthways and scoop out centre into a bowl. Mix with mushrooms and relish and pile back into potato shell. Return to oven for 10 minutes. Shred cabbage and grate carrot. Blend salad dressing with yogurt and mix with vegetables. Serve coleslaw with baked potato. Follow with banana.

Snack 1 ☐	*1 small packet corn snacks, any flavour* *25g/1oz Edam or Tendale cheese*

Snack 2 ☐	*1 individual muesli or fruit and nut bar* *1 medium banana*

☐ If you completed the day without cheating at all, tick here and move on to Day 23.

☐ If you cheated, do a 'Saintly Day' tomorrow (page 253) instead of the set menu.

☐ If you do not eat one meal or snack that you are allowed, tick this box and save up for a 'Naughty Day'. When you have two ticks saved, you can do any of the Thoroughly Naughty Day's Menus *instead* of your next day's diet.

Exercise Day 22

MORNING ☐ Repeat Exercise 1: 5 times

☐ Repeat Exercise 3: 5 times circling left and right with right foot

☐ Repeat Exercise 3: 5 times circling left and right with right foot
5 times circling left and right with left foot

☐ Repeat Exercise 4: touch the floor 15 times

☐ Repeat Exercise 5: bend to left and right 15 times

☐ Repeat Exercise 6: circle to left 15 times
circle to right 15 times
Repeat Exercise 7: criss-cross 20 times

☐ Repeat Exercise 8: stretch 5 times

☐ Repeat Exercise 9: touch left foot and sit up
touch right foot and sit up 15 times

☐ Repeat Exercise 10: floor-walk to wall and back 5 times

Exercise 11 ☐ Lie on stomach. Place hands under forehead with palms on floor and rest for a few minutes. Move hands down beneath shoulders, palms still down and fingers touching. Rest forehead on floor then slowly raise head and trunk by pushing down with hands on the floor. Keeping legs straight on floor arch spine and tilt head back. Hold for the count of 10. Slowly lower yourself back to floor. Rest.

LUNCHTIME ☐ Walk for 26 minutes marking your position 6 minutes from your starting point. Turn and briskly walk to your marked position in 16 minutes, then jog the final stretch.

EVENING ☐ Run to top of stairs and down again 4 times. Jog for 10 minutes.

Or ☐ Jog for 20 minutes:
1st 5-minute jog
2nd 5-minute jog
3rd 5-minute jog
4th 5-minute jog

Then ☐ Skip 175 times.

Bedtime Relaxer ☐

Beauty Shopping List Week 4

The number of items you will require depends on your skin type and problems. Check through the week's treatments and write down the products you need to purchase.

Ammonia	Face pack	Nail clippers or
Baby oil	Hand lotion	scissors
Body lotion	Lemon juice	Nail polish
Buffing paste	Make-up sponge	Nail polish remover
Cleanser	Manicure stick	Pumice stone
Cotton wool	Medicated cover-up	Razor
Cuticle cream	stick	Salt
Depilatory cream	Medicated soap	10-volume peroxide
Depilatory wax	Medicated talc	Toner
Emery boards	Moisturizer	Waterproof emery
Eyebrow tweezers		paper

Beauty Day 22

A blemish may loom large to you but go unnoticed by anyone else, unless you point it out. Spots, scars, discoloured patches can all be camouflaged.

Spots
A crop of spots can be hidden while they are being treated with a medicated cover-up. These are available from chemists in liquid or cream form. Choose a colour which matches your skin.

The odd spot may have a raised head. On page 42, Day 4, you can read how to relieve it. Meanwhile, disguise it with a medicated spot stick, rather like a lipstick but in a skin toning shade.

Veins
Tiny veins are mentioned on page 28, Day 2. They can be hidden with an opaque tinted fluid or cream which should be applied with a very light touch. Thicker stick make-up can be used but a little of this should be softened by warming in the palm of the hand and then applied with fingertips. Match the colour to your natural skin tone but opt for beige, rather than a rosy shade. Fingerprint on and powder over. For a more covering effect, dab on colour, wait for a minute or two, then dab on some more. Stroke away the colour carefully at edges to blend in with your skin. It may work better if you powder between applications. By experimenting you will be able to judge.

Freckles, 'liver' spots and moles
These can be made to disappear beneath the same kind of camouflage as you would use for veins.

Scars
Scars are sometimes pitted. They can be built up to skin level by working in a thick cream or make-up stick with your finger or a spatula. There are products formulated for coping with skin which is darkly stained or extensively pitted. Ask to speak to the dispensing chemist, consult your doctor or contact the dermatological unit of your nearest hospital.

Dark circles under the eyes
These will soften if you apply a very pale cream, white, or tinted fluid. Apply lightener then fingerprint your normal foundation over the top.

Skin too rosy?
Opaque foundation will cool it. Use a stick or 'pancake' make-up and apply with a small flat sponge. Or you could use a piece of cotton wool. Dip sponge or cotton wool in tepid water, squeeze it out so that it is just moist, and polish colour lightly over face. Follow the directions on page 149, Day 18. Finish with a green-tinted face powder which will cool a high colour.

Today's special treatment
If you have any blemishes, give our cover-up tactics a try. You can adapt them to hide blemishes on arms and legs if the area will not rub against clothing.

Eyebrows ☐ Check eyebrows for straggling hairs which may be sprouting again and tweezer them away. Recap, page 98, Day 12.

Move gracefully ☐ Keep moving gracefully. Re read our blueprint for beautiful movers on page 74, Day 8.

Cleanse, tone, moisturize ☐ Cleanse, tone and moisturize your face in the morning and at night.

Hair livener ☐ Massage scalp, see page 61, Day 7, but omit oil.

Shopping Checklist Day 23

Choose your meals, then write in by each relevant item the amount you require.

Amount required	*Amount required*	*Amount required*
Fruit and Vegetables	Edam or Tendale cheese	Low-calorie tartare sauce
Cauliflower	Eggs	Marmalade or jam
Cucumber	Low-fat natural yogurt	Mustard
Leek		Salt and pepper
Lettuce	Low-fat spread	Tomato purée
Mushrooms	Parmesan cheese	Worcestershire sauce
Onion	Skimmed milk	
Tomatoes	**Grocery**	
Watercress	Bran breakfast cereal	
Banana	Crispbreads	
Pears	Currant bun	
Strawberries or raspberries	Dried onion flakes	
Frozen Foods	French bread	
Fish cakes	Fruit in low-calorie syrup or water	
Rice, peas and mushrooms	Low-calorie soup	
Runner beans	Oil-free French dressing	
Strawberries or raspberries	Raisins or sultanas	
Meat, Poultry and Fish	Tuna in brine	
Streaky bacon	Wholemeal bread	
Dairy Produce/Eggs	**Store Cupboard**	
Butter or margarine	Chicken stock cube	
	Cornflour	
Cheese spread		

Diet Day 23

☐ *275ml/½ pint skimmed milk or reconstituted low-fat powdered milk*

BREAKFAST/SUPPER MEAL

Either ☐ *2 eggs, size 3, scrambled with 15ml/1 tablespoon skimmed milk (extra to allowance); 1 tomato, grilled without fat*

Or ☐ *25g/1oz any bran breakfast cereal; 60ml/4 level tablespoons low-fat natural yogurt; 1 pear*

Or ☐ *2 small slices wholemeal bread, 25g/1oz each; 10ml/2 level teaspoons low-fat spread; 10ml/2 level teaspoons marmalade or jam*

LIGHT MEAL

Either to eat at home **Soup, Fish Cakes plus Fruit**

☐ *1 can low-calorie soup, any variety* — *15ml/1 level tablespoon low calorie tartare sauce*
2 fish cakes, 50g/2oz each — *227g/8oz can fruit salad or*
50g/2oz runner beans — *peaches or pears in low-calorie syrup or water*

Heat soup and serve first. Grill fish cakes without added fat and serve with boiled beans and tartare sauce. Finish with fruit.

Or to take to work **Rice and Tuna Salad**

☐ *Half a 227g/8oz packet frozen rice, peas and mushrooms* — *2 tomatoes*
100g/3½oz can tuna in brine — *30ml/2 tablespoons oil-free French dressing*

Boil rice and vegetables as instructed on packet. Drain. Drain and chop tuna and chop tomatoes. Add to rice with oil-free French dressing and take to work in a container.

Or if you prefer to eat vegetarian **Soup and Banana Sandwich**

☐ *1 can low-calorie soup, any variety* — *1 medium banana*
50g/2oz French bread or 2 small slices wholemeal bread, 25g/1oz each — *30ml/2 tablespoons raisins or sultanas*

Heat soup and serve first. Cut French bread in half. Mash banana with raisins or sultanas and spread on top of bread.

*Either an
easy recipe*
**Salad plus
Cheese on
Toast**

Cucumber and lettuce
Onion and watercress
15ml/1 tablespoon oil-free
　French dressing
50g/2oz Edam or Tendale
　cheese

Dash Worcestershire sauce
15ml/1 tablespoon skimmed
　milk
Pinch dry mustard
2 small slices wholemeal
　bread, 25g/1oz each

Make a green salad of as much cucumber, lettuce, onion and
watercress as you wish and serve as a starter sprinkled
with oil-free French dressing. Grate the cheese and mix
with Worcestershire sauce, milk and mustard. Toast bread
on one side. Spread the other side with cheese mixture and
grill until browned.

---

*Or a keen
cook's recipe*
**Mushroom Soup,
Cauliflower
and Leek
Cheese plus
Fruit**

50g/2oz mushrooms
1 chicken stock cube
275ml/½ pint water
Pinch dried onion flakes
Salt and pepper
1 medium leek
175g/6oz cauliflower
5ml/1 level teaspoon butter
　or margarine

15ml/1 level tablespoon
　cornflour
200ml/7floz skimmed milk
1 rasher streaky bacon
10ml/2 level teaspoons
　grated Parmesan cheese
75g/3oz strawberries or
　raspberries, fresh or frozen
30ml/2 tablespoons low-fat
　natural yogurt

Finely slice mushrooms and put into a pan with stock cube,
water and onion flakes. Cover and simmer for 15 minutes.
Season to taste and serve as a starter. Slice and wash leek.
Break cauliflower into florets. Boil both together for about
10 minutes until tender. Drain and put into a small
ovenproof dish. Melt the butter in a small pan. Mix the
cornflour and skimmed milk until smooth and pour onto the
butter, stirring constantly. Bring to the boil, then season.
Grill bacon until crisp. Pour sauce over the vegetables,
sprinkle with cheese and grill to brown. Top with bacon
pieces. Follow with berries and yogurt.

Snack 1

1 currant bun, 50g/1¾oz
10ml/2 level teaspoons low-
　fat spread

1 small banana

Snack 2

20ml/4 teaspoons
　Worcestershire sauce
60ml/4 tablespoons low-fat
　natural yogurt
10ml/2 teaspoons tomato
　purée

2.5ml/½ teaspoon prepared
　mustard
Raw vegetables of your choice
2 crispbreads
2 triangles cheese spread

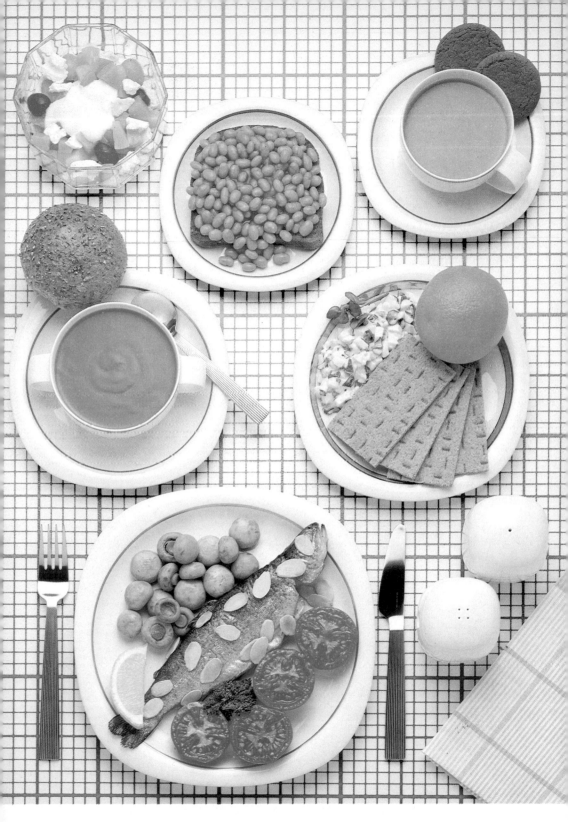

An easy menu for Day 11 could consist of Beans on Toast, Egg Crispbreads, an Orange, Trout and Almonds, Fruit and Meringue, Hot Chocolate and Biscuits and Soup and Roll.

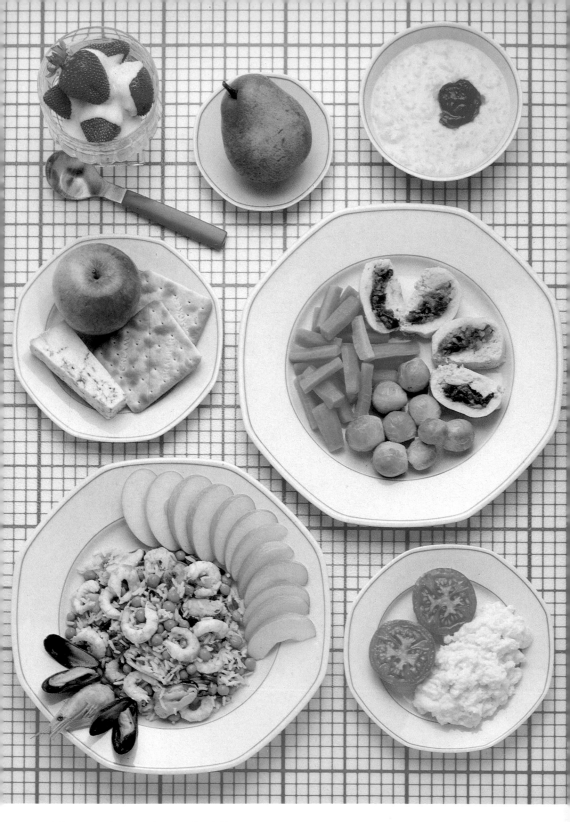

A keen cook may choose the following from Day 17: Scrambled Egg and Tomato, Paella and Apple, Prune Stuffed Chicken, Strawberries and Yogurt, Cheese Crackers and an Apple, Creamed Rice Pudding and a Pear.

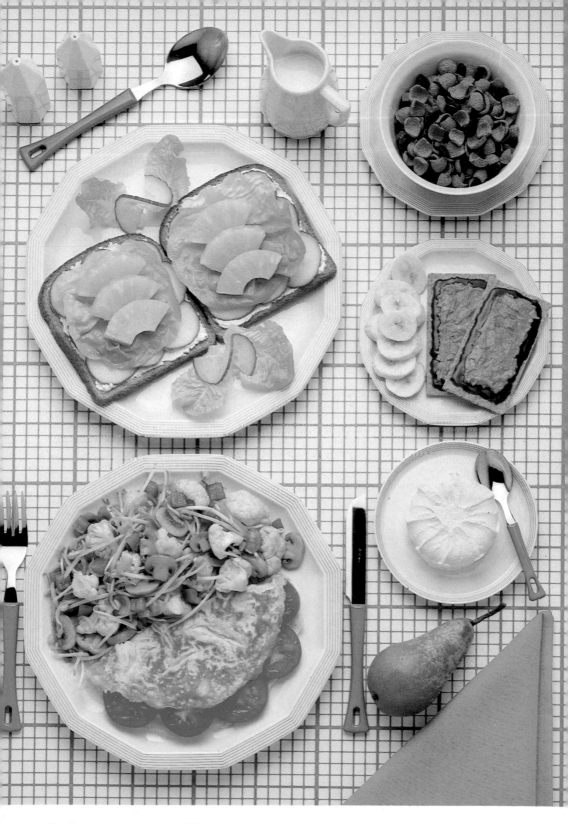

Prefer to eat vegetarian? Day 24 menu choices include: Bran Cereal and Raisins, Cheese and Pineapple Open Sandwich, Omelette and Crunchy Vegetables plus a Pear, Ice Cream, Peanut Butter Crispbreads and a Banana.

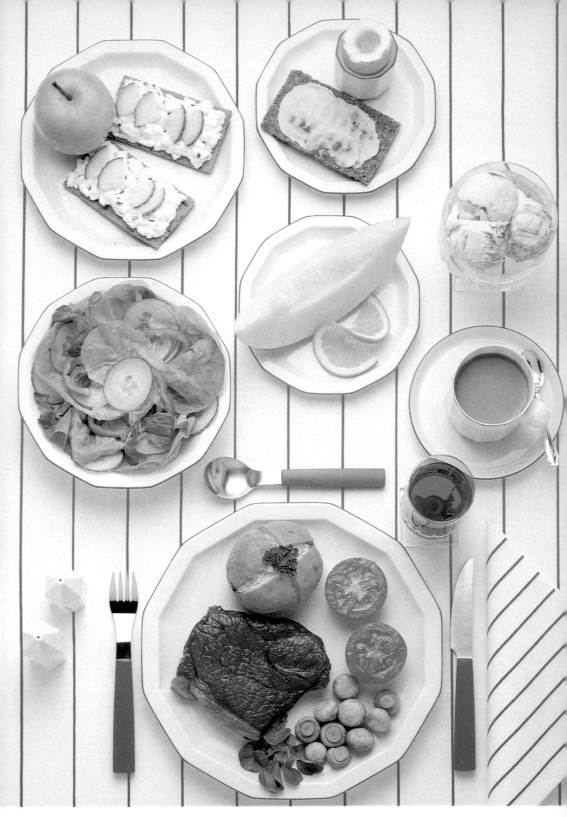

Need to eat out occasionally? Save up for a naughty day and you can enjoy a three-course steak bar meal with wine, plus two light meals — Egg and Crispbread and

Cottage Cheese Crispbreads and an Apple.

Photography/Martin Brigdale.
Stylist/Gina Carminati
Dishes Harrods and Rosenthal;
Cutlery Harrods and David Mellor

Mix together Worcestershire sauce, yogurt, tomato purée and mustard and use it as a dip for vegetables. Spread crispbreads with cheese spread.

☐ If you completed the day without cheating at all, tick here and move on to Day 24.

☐ If you cheated, do a 'Saintly Day' tomorrow (page 253) instead of the set menu.

☐ If you do not eat one meal or snack that you are allowed, tick this box and save up for a 'Naughty Day'. When you have two ticks saved, you can do any of the Thoroughly Naughty Day's Menus *instead* of your next day's diet.

Exercise Day 23

MORNING

☐ Repeat Exercise 1: 5 times

☐ Repeat Exercise 2: 5 times to right
5 times to left

☐ Repeat Exercise 3: 5 times circling left and right with right foot
5 times circling left and right with left foot

☐ Repeat Exercise 4: touch the floor 15 times

☐ Repeat Exercise 5: bend to left and right 15 times

☐ Repeat Exercise 6: circle to left 15 times
circle to right 15 times

☐ Repeat Exercise 7: criss-cross 20 times

☐ Repeat Exercise 8: stretch 5 times

☐ Repeat Exercise 9: touch left foot and sit up
touch right foot and sit up 15 times

☐ Repeat Exercise 10: floor-walk to wall and back 5 times

☐ Repeat Exercise 11: arch spine and lower twice

LUNCHTIME ☐ Walk for 27 minutes, marking your position 7 minutes from your starting point. Turn and briskly walk to your marked place in 16 minutes, then jog the final stretch.

EVENING ☐ Run to top of stairs and down again 4 times. Jog for 10 minutes.

Or ☐ Jog for 20 minutes:
1st 5-minute jog
2nd 5-minute jog
3rd 5-minute jog
4th 5-minute jog

Then ☐ Skip 200 times.
If you cannot manage this number of skips all at once, take a break halfway.

Bedtime Relaxer ☐

Beauty Day 23

Some people have a talent for putting things away and knowing where to find them. They have the answer to all emergencies: needle and thread, nail polish remover or whatever — they can put their hands on them at a moment's notice. *They* never break *their* nails in a scramble for lost belongings. They have a distinct advantage. They may not be more beautiful than those who are slap dash or forgetful. They may not be happier, more lovable or loving, but they save themselves a lot of hassle — and it can show!

No mussed hair, no chipped nail polish, no air of frantic defensiveness: 'What's going to hit me next?' For anyone who longs to swap muddle for method, here are a few basic guidelines:

* Keep the things you use regularly where you can find them. Pack away, give away or throw away any others. Do you possess clothes you haven't worn during the last 6 months? Will you *ever* wear them? Ask yourself if it's worth the clutter of keeping anything which might 'come in handy', especially if it is outdated and does nothing for you.

* Chase things back into their place. Put tights and small items in see-through plastic bags before tucking away.

* Dredge handbag or tote bag frequently. Carry only essentials. Restrict yourself to one bag but ensure that it's large enough. Why buy a tiny, purse-size bag if you have to lug books or a packed lunch in an unglamorous plastic carrier?

* Select the outfit you intend to wear each day the night before, with an alternative in mind in case the weather changes. Leave nothing to chance with spare tights, nail file, nail polish ready in case of accidents. Fight the impulse to wear a new outfit unless you have worked out the right accessories beforehand.

* Buying new clothes hangers? Choose various colours. Keep one colour for trousers and another for dresses, to help you locate clothes in your wardrobe quickly.

* Have make-up at the ready — pencils sharpened, sponges washed, cotton wool divided into useable pieces. Keep a spare kit at work: hairbrush, cleanser, toner, moisturizer, base, talc, blusher, eye pencil, mascara, lip colour.

Today's special treatment

Clear cupboards and reorganize clothes drawers. If some of your clothes are now too big for you, take them in or throw them out. Here is how to take in a pair of jeans:

A. *Remove centre-back belt loop-carrier and set aside. Unpick waistband 3 inches either side of centre-back seam. Unpick centre-back seam to within 4 inches of crotch.*

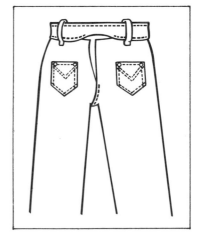

B. *With right sides of fabric together (easier if you turn jeans inside out), tack a giant dart up centre-back seam, taking required amount off at waist and tapering to nothing at crotch. Stitch twice for extra strength. Fold waistband in half, right sides of fabric together, at centre-back and make a seam so that waistband fits reduced jeans. Stitch twice.*

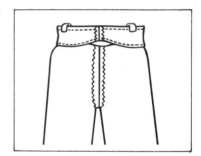

C. *Trim away spare fabric to leave ⅝ths of an inch. Press seams open and neaten by oversewing or zig-zag stitch.*

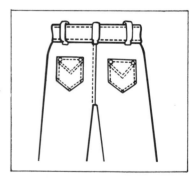

D. *Now top-stitch centre-back seam in contrast thread to match other top-stitching on jeans (use a thicker thread, such as buttonhole twist, and a large stitch). Re-fit unpicked waistband area; tack into position and top-stitch. Replace belt loop-carrier to cover centre-back waistband seam.*

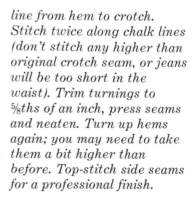

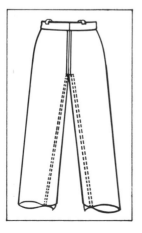

E. *If jeans now fit at waist but are too baggy on the legs, take them in as follows. Unpick hems. Try on jeans inside out and pin a new hem width of 13 to 14 inches on each inside leg. Use more pins to fit jeans snuggly at calf, knee and thigh. Remove jeans carefully; lay them flat. With a ruler and chalk, join up pin positions in a straight line from hem to crotch. Stitch twice along chalk lines (don't stitch any higher than original crotch seam, or jeans will be too short in the waist). Trim turnings to ⅝ths of an inch, press seams and neaten. Turn up hems again; you may need to take them a bit higher than before. Top-stitch side seams for a professional finish.*

Cleanse, tone, moisturize	☐	Cleanse, tone and moisturize your face in the morning and at night.
Hair livener	☐	For dry hair only: massage scalp, see page 61, Day 7, but omit oil.
Spotty back?	☐	Soak in warm bath; scrub back with medicated soap, dry and dab with diluted antiseptic. Dust with medicated talc.
Pedicure	☐	Repeat pedicure from page 81, Day 9.
Body massage	☐	Repeat the body massage from page 29, Day 2.

Shopping Checklist Day 24

Choose your meals, then write in by each relevant item the amount you require.

Amount required	*Amount required*	*Amount required*
Fruit and Vegetables	Eggs	Yeast extract
Bean sprouts	Low-fat natural	
Brussels sprouts	yogurt	
Cauliflower	Low-fat spread	
Courgettes	Skimmed milk	
Cucumber	**Grocery**	
Green pepper	Bran breakfast cereal	
Lettuce	Crispbreads	
Mushrooms	Peanut butter	
Onions	Pineapple canned in	
Spring onions	low-calorie syrup	
Tomatoes	Prunes	
Apple	Raisins or sultanas	
Banana	Sweetcorn	
Orange	Wholemeal bread	
Pear	**Store Cupboard**	
Frozen Foods	Chutney	
Brussels sprouts	Cranberry sauce or	
Courgettes	jelly	
Ice cream	Mint sauce or jelly	
Sweetcorn	Oil	
Meat, Poultry and Fish	Rosemary	
Loin lamb chop	Salt and pepper	
Streaky bacon	Soy sauce	
Dairy Produce/Eggs	Stock cube	
Curd cheese	Tomato purée	

Diet Day 24

275ml/½ pint skimmed milk or reconstituted low-fat powdered milk

BREAKFAST/SUPPER MEAL

Either

1 slice wholemeal bread, 40g/1½oz; 1 egg, size 3; 5ml/1 level teaspoon low-fat spread
Dip bread into beaten egg and fry in a non-stick pan greased with low-fat spread.

Or

25g/1oz any bran breakfast cereal; 75ml/5 level tablespoons skimmed milk; 30ml/2 level tablespoons raisins or sultanas

Or

2 tomatoes, grilled without fat; 2 rashers streaky bacon, well grilled; 1 small slice wholemeal bread, 25g/1oz

LIGHT MEAL

Either to eat at home
Curd Cheese and Pineapple Open Sandwich

2 slices wholemeal bread, 40g/1½oz each	2 rings pineapple canned in low-calorie syrup
50g/2oz curd cheese	Lettuce and cucumber

Spread bread slices with curd cheese. Add lettuce and cucumber and top with pineapple.

Or to take to work
Cheese and Chutney Sandwich plus Fruit Salad

2 small slices wholemeal bread, 25g/1oz each	2 tomatoes
	1 orange
25g/1oz curd or cottage cheese	2 rings pineapple canned in low-calorie syrup

15ml/1 level tablespoon chutney

Spread one slice of bread with cheese and the other with chutney and sandwich together. Take tomatoes whole to eat with sandwich. Peel and slice orange and mix with chopped pineapple. Take to work in a separate container.

MAIN MEAL

Either an easy recipe
Grilled Lamb Chop and Vegetables plus Fruit

150g/5oz lamb loin chop	15ml/1 tablespoon mint sauce or jelly
115g/4oz Brussels sprouts, fresh or frozen	1 medium apple or pear
115g/4oz sweetcorn, frozen or canned	

Discard all visible fat from chop and grill well. Boil sprouts and sweetcorn. Serve chop with vegetables and mint sauce. Follow with fruit.

Or a keen cook's recipe **Braised Chop with Ratatouille plus Prunes**

150g/5oz lamb loin chop
1 small onion
150g/5oz courgettes, fresh or frozen
2 tomatoes
15ml/1 level tablespoon cranberry sauce or jelly
150ml/¼ pint water
½ stock cube
5ml/1 level teaspoon tomato purée
Rosemary
6 soaked prunes
60ml/4 tablespoons low-fat natural yogurt

Discard all visible fat from chop. Slice onion, courgettes and tomatoes and place in a small ovenproof casserole. Place chop on top and spread with cranberry sauce or jelly. Add water, stock cube, tomato purée and a good pinch of rosemary. Cover and cook at 180°C/350°F, gas mark 4, for about 1 hour until the meat is tender. Follow with prunes and yogurt.

Or if you prefer to eat vegetarian **Omelet and Crunchy Vegetables**

10ml/2 teaspoons oil
150g/5oz cauliflower
115g/4oz mushrooms
½ green pepper
2 spring onions or ½ small onion
1 fresh or canned tomato
115g/4oz bean sprouts
5ml/1 level teaspoon Soy sauce
Salt and pepper
2 eggs, size 3
30ml/2 tablespoons skimmed milk
5ml/1 level teaspoon low-fat spread
1 small apple or pear

Heat oil in a non-stick frying pan. Cut cauliflower into small florets; slice mushrooms; chop pepper and spring onion. Slice tomato. Heat oil in a non-stick frying pan and stir-fry cauliflower for 3 minutes. Add mushrooms, pepper and spring onion and cook for a further 3 minutes, stirring. Add bean sprouts and Soy sauce and cook for 2 minutes. Season to taste and keep warm. Beat eggs with milk and seasoning. Melt low-fat spread in a non-stick omelet pan and brush over surface. Add beaten egg. Cook until mixture is almost set then add tomato slices and fold in half. Serve with crunchy vegetables. Follow with apple or pear.

Snack 1

1 individual ice cream, any flavour

Snack 2 ☐
2 crispbreads   *15ml/1 level tablespoon*
10ml/2 teaspoons yeast   *peanut butter*
extract   *1 small banana*

☐ If you completed the day without cheating at all, tick here and move on to Day 25.

☐ If you cheated, do a 'Saintly Day' tomorrow (page 253) instead of the set menu.

☐ If you do not eat one meal or snack that you are allowed, tick this box and save up for a 'Naughty Day'. When you have two ticks saved, you can do any of the Thoroughly Naughty Day's Menus *instead* of your next day's diet.

Exercise Day 24

MORNING ☐ Repeat Exercise 1: 5 times

☐ Repeat Exercise 2: 5 times to right
5 times to left

☐ Repeat Exercise 3: 5 times circling left and right with right foot
5 times circling left and right with left foot

☐ Repeat Exercise 4: touch the floor 15 times

☐ Repeat Exercise 5: bend to left and right 15 times

☐ Repeat Exercise 6: circle to left 15 times
circle to right 15 times

☐ Repeat Exercise 7: criss-cross 20 times

☐ Repeat Exercise 8: stretch 5 times

☐ Repeat Exercise 9: touch left foot and sit up
touch right foot, and sit up 15 times

☐ Repeat Exercise 10: floor-walk to wall and back 5 times

☐ Repeat Exercise 11: arch spine and lower 3 times

LUNCHTIME ☐ Walk for 28 minutes, marking your position 8 minutes from your starting point. Turn and briskly walk to your marked place in 16 minutes, then jog the final stretch.

EVENING ☐ Run to top of stairs and down again 4 times. Jog for 10 minutes.

Or ☐ Jog for 20 minutes:
1st 5-minute jog
2nd 5-minute jog
3rd 5-minute jog
4th 5-minute jog

Then ☐ Skip 200 times.

☐ Then do the following skipping variation 25 times:

Jump-skip ☐ Bring rope over head and jump with both feet together. Then bring rope over head and jump with feet apart. Continue to jump with feet alternately together and then apart.

Bedtime Relaxer ☐

Beauty Day 24

Scent is never quite the same on any two people, and the fragrance which wafts so tantalizingly when your friend uses it may not be as exciting on you. Scent needs time to reveal its true essence. It takes time to develop on your skin, where oils and other substances can make it smell quite different from the aroma you sniff straight from the bottle. The first impression can be quite overpowering, perhaps a little sharp. Then skin temperature begins to take effect, defining some ingredients, diffusing others, giving fragrance a more full-bodied quality. It mellows and slowly begins to fade. There are so many ingredients which are used to blend perfume it is almost impossible to categorize any particular variety. A scent which is basically floral may have underlying woody notes: for example, patchouli or sandalwood; or a woody scent may be laced with rose or heady jasmine. Natural ingredients may combine with aromatic chemicals to produce a perfume with a personality all of its own. Some perfumes have as many as a hundred different ingredients.

How do you choose a scent?
Frankly, the best way is to follow your nose.

Sampling
Try sampling before buying. Dab a drop on the inside of your wrist and leave it for 15 minutes. Only then will you be able to take in the full bouquet.

Take your time
Test more than 1 fragrance before finally deciding, but no more than 3 at a time, or you will get confused.

Fragrance facts

* Scent may react with a sharper note on dryer skin. Try smoothing on a touch of almond oil beforehand.

* Warmth 'brings out' scent. Body warmth works extra effectively on pulse points: wrist, inside elbows, throat.

* Scents come in various strengths. Perfume concentrate is the most expensive and should be used sparingly. A 'skin perfume' is normally a diluted version, although in some cases this, too, can be highly concentrated. 'Toilet water' is a scent diluted with alcohol and 'cologne' implies the

lightest mix of all. Splash or spray on as much of these as you like.

* Store scent away from light and keep it cool. Atomizers can be kept in the refrigerator when the weather is hot. This way you get less evaporation and a refreshingly ice-cool spray.

Today's special treatment
Repeat the home facial, from page 37, Day 3. Follow it with a face pack, page 43, Day 4 or page 111, Day 14. Moisturize afterwards if skin has a natural tendency to be dry. Leave off make-up for at least an hour.

Hair livener   Massage scalp, see page 61, Day 7, but omit oil.

Elbows   Still rough or discoloured? Mix lemon juice with a little salt and rub in. Rinse off after 5 to 10 minutes and apply body lotion.

Dinginess?   Blend hand cream with 6 drops of 10-volume peroxide and smooth into dingy areas on thighs and under arms.

Goosepimples?   Lather goosepimply areas with a soft brush. Splash with cold water, pat dry and rub in cream or body lotion.

Neck treat   Repeat treatment from page 49, Day 5 to keep neck supple.

Remove unwanted hair   Check for regrowth and treat unwanted hair (see page 86, Day 10).

Shopping Checklist Day 25

Choose your meals, then write in by each relevant item the amount you require.

Amount required	*Amount required*	*Amount required*
Fruit and Vegetables	Pork fillet	Wholemeal bread
Broccoli	Streaky bacon	**Store Cupboard**
Carrot	**Dairy Produce/Eggs**	Artificial sweetener
Celery	Camembert	Dried mixed herbs
Garlic	Edam or Tendale	Salt and pepper
Mushrooms	cheese	Sugar
Onions	Eggs	
Spinach	Low-fat fruit	
Tomatoes	yogurt	
Apple	Low-fat natural	
Banana	yogurt	
Kiwi fruit	Low-fat spread	
Orange	Skimmed milk	
Pear	**Grocery**	
Strawberries	Bran breakfast cereal	
Frozen Foods	Butter beans	
Broccoli	Canned tomatoes	
Kipper fillets	Cream crackers or	
Peas and carrots	water biscuits	
Spinach	Crispbreads	
Strawberries	Custard powder	
Sweetcorn	Ground rice	
Water ice or	Pineapple canned in	
ice cream	natural juice or	
Meat, Poultry and Fish	low-calorie syrup	
Kipper fillets	Sweetcorn	

Diet Day 25

☐ 275ml/½ pint skimmed milk or reconstituted low-fat powdered milk

BREAKFAST/SUPPER MEAL

Either ☐ 2 tomatoes, grilled without fat; 2 rashers streaky bacon, well grilled; 1 small slice wholemeal bread, 25g/1oz

Or ☐ 1 egg, size 3, boiled; 1 small slice wholemeal bread, 25g/1oz; 5ml/1 level teaspoon low-fat spread

Or ☐ 25g/1oz any bran breakfast cereal; 60ml/4 level tablespoons low-fat natural yogurt; 1 small apple

LIGHT MEAL

Either to eat
at home
Kippers and
Tomatoes

☐ 75g/3oz kipper fillets   5ml/1 level teaspoon low-fat
2 tomatoes   spread
1 small slice wholemeal   1 small pear or orange
   bread, 25g/1oz

Poach kipper fillets in a little water. Grill the tomatoes without fat. Serve kippers and tomatoes with bread scraped with low-fat spread. Follow with pear or orange.

Or to take
to work
Kipper Pâté
and
Crispbreads
plus Fruit

☐ 50g/2oz kipper fillet   Freshly ground black pepper
1 small onion   2 tomatoes
5ml/1 level teaspoon low-fat   2 crispbreads
   spread   1 medium apple or pear

Cook kipper fillet as above and allow to cool. Chop onion, boil for 5 minutes, then drain. Blend together kipper, onion, low-fat spread and pepper (either in a liquidizer, food processor or by hand). Take pâté to work in a little pot and eat with tomatoes and crispbreads. Follow with fruit.

Or if you
prefer to eat
vegetarian
Vegetarian
Hot Pot plus
Banana

☐ 1 medium carrot   Pinch dried mixed herbs
¼ onion   Salt and pepper
1 stick celery   213g/7½oz can butter beans
227g/8oz can tomatoes   1 banana
½ clove garlic

Peel and slice carrot, chop onion and celery. Place

vegetables in a saucepan with tomatoes. Crush garlic and add to the pan with herbs. Cover and simmer for 15-20 minutes until carrots are cooked. Drain beans, add to saucepan and heat gently. Follow with banana.

MAIN MEAL

Either a quick recipe **Roast Pork Fillet plus Pineapple and Ice**

1 rasher streaky bacon
75g/3oz pork fillet
115g/4oz peas and carrots, frozen
50g/2oz sweetcorn, frozen or canned

2 rings pineapple, canned in natural juice or low-calorie syrup
50g/2oz water ice or 25g/1oz vanilla ice cream

Wrap streaky bacon round pork fillet and place them on a piece of foil. Make into a parcel and bake at 180°C/350°F, gas mark 4, for 1 hour. Boil vegetables and serve with pork fillet and bacon. Serve pineapple with water ice or ice cream.

Or a keen cook's recipe **Pork Fillet with Mushroom Stuffing plus Pineapple Custard**

115g/4oz pork fillet
1 small onion
50g/2oz mushrooms
60ml/4 level tablespoons fresh breadcrumbs
Salt and pepper
15ml/1 tablespoon skimmed milk
115g/4oz broccoli

115g/4oz carrots
2 rings pineapple, canned in natural juice or low-calorie syrup
10ml/2 level teaspoons custard powder
150ml/¼ pint skimmed milk
5ml/1 level teaspoon sugar
Artificial sweetener, optional

Put pork on a square of foil. Chop onion and slice mushrooms and poach them in a very little water for 5 minutes. Drain and mix onion and mushrooms with breadcrumbs, seasoning and skimmed milk. Spread mixture on pork fillet and fold foil over to enclose food completely. Bake at 180°C/350°F, gas mark 4, for about 1 hour or until pork is tender. Boil broccoli and carrots and serve with pork. Cut pineapple into pieces and put in a serving bowl. Make custard in the usual way. Add a little artificial sweetener if necessary. Pour custard over pineapple. Cover with greaseproof paper to stop skin forming and chill well. Serve after pork.

Or if you prefer to eat vegetarian
Baked Cheesy Spinach and Pineapple Rice

☐

175g/6oz spinach, frozen or lightly boiled fresh
1 egg, size 3
45ml/3 tablespoons skimmed milk
25g/1oz Edam or Tendale cheese
Salt and pepper
30ml/2 level tablespoons ground rice
150ml/¼ pint skimmed milk
5ml/1 level teaspoon sugar
1 pineapple ring

Chop spinach and press out any excess moisture. Beat egg and milk together, then stir in grated cheese. Stir egg mixture into the spinach and season to taste. Pour into a lightly greased small ovenproof dish. Bake at 180°C/350°F, gas mark 4, for 30 minutes. Serve hot. Put rice and milk into a small pan and bring to the boil, stirring continuously. Simmer for 5 minutes until thickened, then stir in sugar. Pour into a serving dish and top with pineapple.

Snack 1 ☐

1 small carton low-fat fruit yogurt
1 kiwi fruit or pear
115g/4oz strawberries, fresh or frozen

Mix fruit with yogurt or eat separately.

Snack 2 ☐

3 cream crackers or large water biscuits
1 individual portion Camembert cheese, 35g/1¼oz

☐ If you completed the day without cheating at all, tick here and move on to Day 26.

☐ If you cheated, do a 'Saintly Day' tomorrow (page 253) instead of the set menu.

☐ If you do not eat one meal or snack that you are allowed, tick this box and save up for a 'Naughty Day'. When you have two ticks saved, you can do any of the Thoroughly Naughty Day's Menus *instead* of your next day's diet.

Exercise Day 25

MORNING ☐ Repeat Exercise 1: 5 times

☐ Repeat Exercise 2: 5 times to right
5 times to left

☐ Repeat Exercise 3: 5 times circling left and right with right foot
5 times circling left and right with left foot

☐ Repeat Exercise 4: touch the floor 15 times

☐ Repeat Exercise 5: bend to left and right 15 times

☐ Repeat Exercise 6: circle to left 15 times
circle to right 15 times

☐ Repeat Exercise 7: criss-cross 20 times

☐ Repeat Exercise 8: stretch 5 times

☐ Repeat Exercise 9: touch left foot and sit up
touch right foot and sit up 15 times

☐ Repeat Exercise 10: floor-walk to wall and back 5 times

☐ Repeat Exercise 11: arch spine and lower 3 times

Exercise 12 ☐ Still lying on floor put arms down by sides and make a fist with hands. Rest chin on floor and pushing down with fists raise left leg as high as you can keeping leg straight. Hold while counting to 5 then slowly lower. Repeat with the right leg. Repeat 4 more times with each leg.

LUNCHTIME ☐ Walk for 29 minutes, marking your position 9 minutes from your starting point. Turn and briskly walk to your marked place in 16 minutes, then jog the final stretch.

EVENING ☐ Run to the top of the stairs and down again 4 times. Jog for 10 minutes.

Or ☐ Jog for 20 minutes:
1st 5-minute jog
2nd 5-minute jog

3rd 5-minute jog
4th 5-minute jog

Run-skip 200 times.

Jump-skip 50 times.

Bedtime Relaxer

Beauty Day 25

Arms so often get neglected. Though plump arms will slim along with the rest of your body as you diet away surplus weight, the underside of the bicep area often needs extra exercise attention in order to avoid a flabby 'undercarriage' when arms are extended. Today's special exercise can help firm up flab on upper arms. Meanwhile, disguise is easy. Sleeves which end just above elbows, or a little below, are decidedly more flattering than sleeveless tops and dresses or small 'cap' sleeves. An overall colour from shoulders downwards gives a leaner look than contrasting top and skirt.

Golden-brown arms tend to look slimmer — or at least prettier — than uncovered areas of white podgy flesh. So a light tan is worth aiming at.

Downy arms? Don't worry
Hair grows in longer strands over arms but goes unnoticed if it's fine and fair. A darker growth shows up less on a tanned skin, and the sun tends to lighten hair; if it doesn't, most chemists sell a bleaching cream to do the same job. For a home-made bleach: 5 drops of household ammonia mixed with 2 tablespoons of 10-volume peroxide. Stroke on with cotton wool. Rinse off with warm water after 7-10 minutes and smooth in hand cream.

Restrict bleaching to twice a week at 2- or 3-day intervals, and the problem should soon fade away.

Today's special treatment
A super-silky treat for arms. You can build it into your Day 2, page 29, massage or practise it separately to tone arms.

Work cream or body lotion into arms with circular movements from wrist to elbow. Circle round elbow with palm. Circle up from elbow to shoulder. Do this arm massage at night, before going to bed.

Windmill waver
for toning

☐ Stand with arms outstretched. Circle arms in one direction 5 times. Reverse the direction and circle 5 more times. Keep the movement slow and measured and make wide circles. Once a day for 2 days and then 2 or 3 times a day.

Cleanse, tone,
moisturize

☐ Cleanse, tone and moisturize your face in the morning and at night.

Hair livener

☐ For dry hair only: massage scalp, see page 61, Day 7, but omit oil.

Spotty back?

☐ Soak in warm bath; scrub back with medicated soap, dry and dab with diluted antiseptic. Dust with medicated talc.

Blackheads?

☐ Repeat steam treatment from page 42, Day 4.

Shopping Checklist Day 26

Choose your meals, then write in by each relevant item the amount you require.

Amount required	*Amount required*	*Amount required*
Fruit and Vegetables	Skimmed milk	Oil-free French
Green beans	**Grocery**	dressing
Mushrooms	Baked beans in	Salt and pepper
Onion	tomato sauce	Sugar
Tomatoes	Bran breakfast cereal	Tomato ketchup
Apple	Branston-type pickle	
Orange or satsuma	Broad beans	
Peach	Corn snack	
Pear	Crispbreads	
Frozen Foods	Dried apricots	
Broad beans	Fruit salad or	
Cod in butter or	fruit cocktail in	
parsley sauce	low-calorie syrup	
Green beans	Instant low-calorie	
Oven or grill chips	soup	
Peas	Instant potato powder	
Sweetcorn	Lemon juice	
Meat, Poultry and Fish	Pasta shells	
Chipolata sausage	Sweetcorn	
Cod cutlet	Wholemeal bap	
Dairy Produce/Eggs	Wholemeal bread	
Cottage cheese	**Store Cupboard**	
Eggs	Low-calorie salad	
Low-fat natural	dressing	
yogurt	Marmalade or jam	
Low-fat spread	Mixed herbs	

Diet Day 26

☐ 275ml/½ pint skimmed milk or reconstituted low-fat powdered milk

BREAKFAST/SUPPER MEAL

Either ☐ 2 eggs, size 3, scrambled with 15ml/1 tablespoon skimmed milk; 1 tomato, grilled without fat

Or ☐ 25g/1oz any bran breakfast cereal; 75ml/5 tablespoons skimmed milk; 2 dried apricots, chopped

Or ☐ 2 small slices wholemeal bread, 25g/1oz each; 10ml/2 level teaspoons low-fat spread; 10ml/2 level teaspoons marmalade or jam

LIGHT MEAL

Either to eat at home
Soup, Sausage and Baked Beans plus Fruit

☐ 1 sachet instant low calorie soup, any flavour
2 beef or pork chipolata sausages

150g/5.3oz can baked beans in tomato sauce
1 peach or pear

Start with soup. Well grill sausages and serve with heated beans. Follow with fruit.

Or to take to work
Sausage and Bean Salad plus Fruit

☐ 25g/1oz pasta shells, raw
1 beef or pork chipolata sausage
50g/2oz broad beans, frozen or canned
15ml/1 level tablespoon low-calorie salad dressing
15ml/1 tablespoon oil-free French dressing

Salt and pepper
2 crispbreads
10ml/2 level teaspoons low-fat spread
1 peach or pear

Boil pasta in salted water and allow to cool. Well grill sausage and cut into slices. Boil beans and drain. Mix pasta, beans and sausage with low-calorie salad dressing and oil-free French dressing and season to taste. Take to work in a plastic container and eat with crispbread scraped with low-fat spread. Follow with fruit.

Or if you prefer to eat vegetarian
Spicy Beans on Toast plus Fruit

150g/5.3oz can baked beans in tomato sauce
15ml/1 level tablespoon Branston-type pickle

1 slice wholemeal bread, 40g/1½oz
1 medium apple

Heat beans and mix with pickle. Serve on toasted bread. Follow with fruit.

To take to work

Make up the bean salad above but use 15g/½oz Cheshire or Cotswold cheese instead of sausage.

MAIN MEAL

Either a quick recipe
Cod in Sauce plus Fruit

1 packet frozen cod in butter or parsley sauce
115g/4oz peas

45ml/3 level tablespoons instant potato powder
1 small orange or satsuma

Cook fish as instructed on packet. Boil peas and make up potato using water. Do not add any butter. Serve cod in sauce with vegetables. Follow with orange.

Or a keen cook's recipe
Herby Cod Cutlet plus Orange Caramel

150g/5oz cod cutlet, bone removed
25g/1oz mushrooms
25g/1oz onion
60ml/4 level tablespoons fresh breadcrumbs
Salt and pepper
5ml/1 teaspoon lemon juice

Pinch mixed herbs
45ml/3 level tablespoons instant potato powder
115g/4oz green beans
1 orange
15ml/1 level tablespoon sugar

Put the cutlet in a square of foil. Slice mushrooms and chop onion. Poach them in a little water for 5 minutes and drain. Mix with breadcrumbs, seasoning and lemon juice. Use to fill cavity in the cutlet. Sprinkle with herbs. Fold foil to enclose fish completely and bake at 180°C/350°F, gas mark 4, for 30 minutes. Mix potato powder with water and boil beans. Serve with herby cod. Dissolve sugar in 15ml/1 tablespoon water. Boil until it goes a dark brown. Remove from heat and add 45ml/3 tablespoons hot water. Return to heat and dissolve. Allow to cool and pour over sliced orange.

Or if you prefer to eat vegetarian
Egg Muffin and Chips

115g/4oz oven or grill chips
½ wholemeal bap
1 egg, size 3
15ml/1 level tablespoon tomato ketchup

15ml/1 level tablespoon low-calorie salad dressing
15ml/1 tablespoon low-fat natural yogurt

Cook chips as instructed on packet. Toast bap. Poach egg in water or a non-stick poacher without fat. Put tomato ketchup, salad dressing and yogurt in a saucepan and heat gently. Place poached egg on bap. Cover with sauce and serve with chips.

Snack 1 ☐ *113g/4oz carton cottage cheese with chives, with onion and peppers or with pineapple*   *1 small packet corn snacks, any flavour*

Snack 2 ☐ *227g/8oz can fruit salad or fruit cocktail in low-calorie syrup*   *30ml/2 tablespoons low-fat natural yogurt* *25g/1oz pasta shells*   *15ml/1 tablespoon low-calorie salad dressing*
Drain fruit. Boil pasta. Drain and mix with fruit. Mix yogurt with salad dressing and add to fruit.

☐ If you completed the day without cheating at all, tick here and move on to Day 27.

☐ If you cheated, do a 'Saintly Day' tomorrow (page 253) instead of the set menu.

☐ If you do not eat one meal or snack that you are allowed, tick this box and save up for a 'Naughty Day'. When you have two ticks saved, you can do any of the Thoroughly Naughty Day's Menus *instead* of your next day's diet.

Exercise Day 26

MORNING ☐ Repeat Exercise 1: 5 times

☐ Repeat Exercise 2: 5 times to right
5 times to left

☐ Repeat Exercise 3: 5 times circling left and right with right foot
5 times circling left and right with left foot

☐ Repeat Exercise 4: touch the floor 15 times

☐ Repeat Exercise 5: bend to left and right 15 times

☐ Repeat Exercise 6: circle to left 15 times
circle to right 15 times

☐ Repeat Exercise 7: criss-cross 20 times

☐ Repeat Exercise 8: stretch 5 times

☐ Repeat Exercise 9: touch left foot and sit up
touch right foot and sit up 15 times

☐ Repeat Exercise 10: floor-walk to wall and back 5 times

☐ Repeat Exercise 11: arch spine and lower 3 times

☐ Repeat Exercise 12: raise left then right leg 10 times

LUNCHTIME ☐ Walk for 30 minutes, marking your position 10 minutes from your starting point. Turn and briskly walk to your marked place in 16 minutes, then jog the final stretch.

EVENING ☐ Run to top of stairs and down again 4 times. Jog for 10 minutes.

Or ☐ Jog for 20 minutes:
1st 5-minute jog   3rd 5-minute jog
2nd 5-minute jog   4th 5-minute jog

Then ☐ Run-skip 200 times.

Then ☐ Jump-skip 100 times.

Bedtime Relaxer ☐

Beauty Day 26

First steps to lovelier legs
Follow our diet to get rid of excess fat and keep working hard at the exercises.

Give legs a longer look

* Because anything pale tends to loom larger, bare legs look leaner when they are tanned. Options are sun, sun beds or the fake tanning lotions. The latter tint skin a few shades darker, and won't wash off but fade gradually. There *are* drawbacks; it's easy to miss a patch of skin and leave a pale stripe. So smooth in very evenly, and be sure to wash your hands very carefully afterwards. The lotion may 'take' more strongly where skin is drier, so rub in body cream a few hours beforehand as a precaution. Legs tend to be dryest over knees and behind ankles.

* Colour-matching shoes and tights give the impression of longer, leaner legs. Opt for a medium to deep tone: smoky brown, olive, navy.

* Wear an open-fronted shoe; no ankle strap to foreshorten legs or draw attention to ankles. An elegantly plain court shoe is the most elongating.

* Choose a medium-high heel, and one that's not too spindly — or legs can look thicker by contrast!

* Experiment to find your ideal hemline. Unless your legs deserve maximum attention, give anything 'mini' a miss; usually, a stopping point just below your knee is most flattering. Long skirts tend to be dumpy-making unless you are tall.

Today's special treatment

Scrutinize legs. Can you grip a handful of flesh? Check for flab this way. Sit, bend your knees and raise your legs. Pat thighs and calves. Does the flesh wobble? Cycling will help you firm these areas. If you don't have a bicycle, try this exercise:

Lie on the floor on your back. Lift legs into the air, keeping them straight. Now do cycling movements in the air for as long as you can. Rest, then repeat the exercise once more.

Check legs for surplus hair and remove if necessary (see page 86, Day 10). Stroke body lotion onto legs. Place hands on either side of your ankles and make circling movements with your fingers. Make long upward strokes to knee, and then more circling movements. Then make upward strokes over thighs.

Cleanse, tone, moisturize

Cleanse, tone and moisturize your face in the morning and at night.

219

Hair livener ☐ Massage scalp, see page 61, Day 7, but omit oil.

Eye soother ☐ Remember that whenever your eyes feel tired, repeat the treatment from page 157, Day 19.

Shopping Checklist Day 27

Choose your meals, then write in by each relevant item the amount you require.

Amount required	*Amount required*	*Amount required*
Fruit and Vegetables	Low-fat spread	**Store Cupboard**
Bean sprouts	Low-fat strawberry	Drinking chocolate
Carrot	yogurt	Garlic salt
Cauliflower	Parmesan cheese	Low-calorie salad
Courgettes	Ricotta or curd	dressing
Cucumber	cheese	Oil-free French
Leek	Skimmed milk	dressing
Lettuce	**Grocery**	Salt and pepper
Onion	Apple sauce	
Potato	Bean sprouts	
Red or white cabbage	Bran breakfast cereal	
Tomatoes	Crispbreads	
Watercress	Crusty roll	
Grapes	Dill pickle or	
Frozen Foods	gherkin	
Courgettes	Gingernut or malted	
Sweetcorn	milk biscuit	
Meat, Poultry and Fish	Ground walnuts	
Chicken	Low-calorie soup	
Chipolata sausages	Raisins	
Corned beef	Sultanas	
Prawns	Sweetcorn	
Dairy Produce/Eggs	Sweet pickle	
Edam or Tendale	White sauce mix	
cheese	Wholemeal bread	
Eggs	Wholewheat pasta	

Diet Day 27

☐ *275ml/½ pint skimmed milk or reconstituted low-fat powdered milk*

BREAKFAST/SUPPER MEAL

Either ☐ *1 slice wholemeal bread, 40g/1½oz; 1 egg, size 3; 5ml/1 level teaspoon low-fat spread*
Dip bread into beaten egg and fry in non-stick pan greased with low-fat spread.

Or ☐ *25g/1oz any bran breakfast cereal; 75ml/5 level tablespoons skimmed milk; 30ml/2 level tablespoons raisins or sultanas*

Or ☐ *2 tomatoes, grilled without fat; 2 beef or pork chipolata sausages, well grilled; 2 small slices wholemeal bread, 25g/1oz each*

LIGHT MEAL

Either to eat at home
Chicken and Vegetables

☐ *225g/8oz chicken leg joint*
50g/2oz sweetcorn, frozen or canned
115g/4oz bean sprouts, fresh or canned
15ml/1 tablespoon apple sauce

Wrap chicken joint in foil and bake in the oven at 200°C/400°F, gas mark 6, for 45 minutes. Boil sweetcorn and bean sprouts and mix together. When chicken is cooked remove and discard skin. Serve chicken with vegetables and apple sauce.

Or to take to work
Chicken and Corn Salad

☐ *50g/2oz cooked chicken meat, skin removed*
50g/2oz sweetcorn, frozen or canned
Cucumber
15ml/1 level tablespoon sultanas
15ml/1 level tablespoon low-calorie salad dressing
2 crispbreads

Cut chicken into bite-size pieces. Cook frozen sweetcorn then drain and cool. Dice about ¼ cucumber. Mix chicken with vegetables and add sultanas and salad dressing. Take to work in a container and eat with crispbreads.

Or if you prefer to eat vegetarian **Cabbage and Carrot Salad with Cheese**

175g/6oz red or white cabbage
50g/2oz carrot
75g/3oz leek or onion
30ml/2 tablespoons oil-free French dressing

15ml/1 tablespoon low-calorie salad dressing
25g/1oz Edam or Tendale cheese
1 crispbread
5ml/1 level teaspoon low-fat spread

Shred cabbage; grate carrot and thinly slice leek or onion. Mix together and add dressing. Toss until thoroughly mixed and add cheese cut into cubes. Serve with crispbread scraped with low-fat spread.

MAIN MEAL

Either a quick recipe **Corned Beef and Potato plus Strawberry Yogurt**

115g/4oz potato
15ml/1 tablespoon skimmed milk
2 tomatoes
50g/2oz corned beef

1 large dill pickle or gherkin
15ml/1 level tablespoon sweet pickle
1 small carton low-fat strawberry yogurt

Boil potato and mash with skimmed milk. Grill tomatoes. Serve with corned beef and pickles. Follow with strawberry yogurt.

Or a keen cook's recipe **Stuffed Courgette plus Grapes**

2 large courgettes
1 small onion
3 tomatoes
115g/4oz peeled prawns
½ packet white sauce mix

150ml/¼ pint skimmed milk
30ml/2 level tablespoons grated Parmesan cheese
115g/4oz cauliflower
115g/4oz grapes

Wash courgettes and boil whole for 10 minutes. Drain and allow to cool. Cut in half lengthways. Scoop out and discard some of the seeds and place courgettes on an ovenproof dish. Boil onion for 5 minutes: drain and chop. Chop tomatoes and mix with onion and prawns. Put into courgette shells. Make up white sauce using skimmed milk and pour over courgettes. Sprinkle on the Parmesan cheese and grill to heat through. Serve with boiled cauliflower. Follow with grapes.

Or if you prefer to eat vegetarian **Pasta in Walnut and Cheese Sauce**

25g/1oz wholewheat pasta
25g/1oz ground walnuts
50g/2oz riccotta or curd cheese
5ml/1 teaspoon Parmesan cheese

Pinch garlic salt, optional
Salt and pepper
Lettuce
Cucumber
Watercress
Onion

Cook pasta as instructed on packet. Mix ground walnuts in

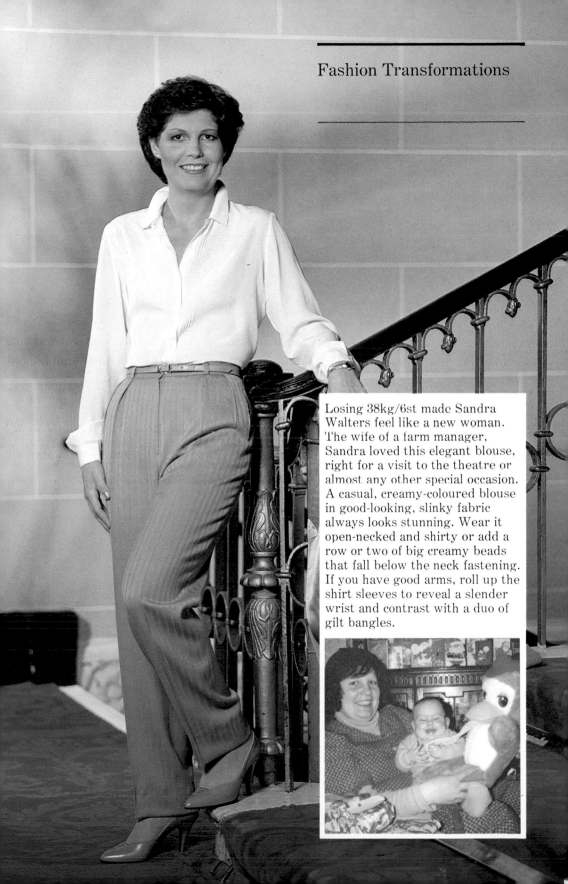

Losing 38kg/6st made Sandra Walters feel like a new woman. The wife of a farm manager, Sandra loved this elegant blouse, right for a visit to the theatre or almost any other special occasion. A casual, creamy-coloured blouse in good-looking, slinky fabric always looks stunning. Wear it open-necked and shirty or add a row or two of big creamy beads that fall below the neck fastening. If you have good arms, roll up the shirt sleeves to reveal a slender wrist and contrast with a duo of gilt bangles.

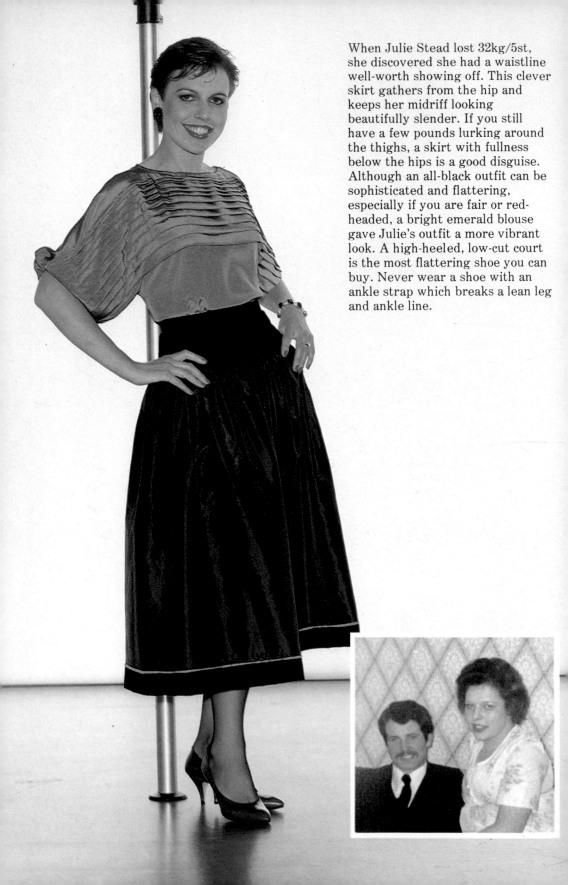

When Julie Stead lost 32kg/5st, she discovered she had a waistline well-worth showing off. This clever skirt gathers from the hip and keeps her midriff looking beautifully slender. If you still have a few pounds lurking around the thighs, a skirt with fullness below the hips is a good disguise. Although an all-black outfit can be sophisticated and flattering, especially if you are fair or red-headed, a bright emerald blouse gave Julie's outfit a more vibrant look. A high-heeled, low-cut court is the most flattering shoe you can buy. Never wear a shoe with an ankle strap which breaks a lean leg and ankle line.

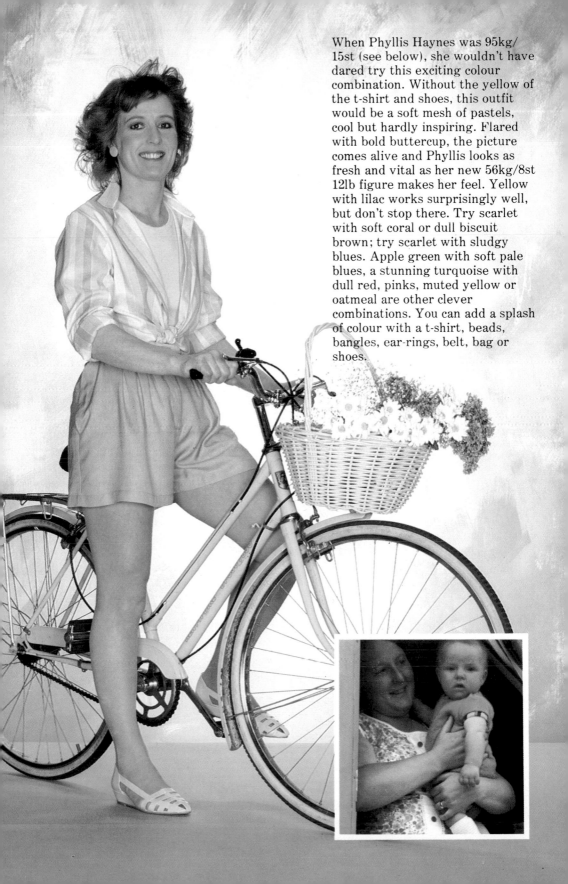

When Phyllis Haynes was 95kg/
15st (see below), she wouldn't have
dared try this exciting colour
combination. Without the yellow of
the t-shirt and shoes, this outfit
would be a soft mesh of pastels,
cool but hardly inspiring. Flared
with bold buttercup, the picture
comes alive and Phyllis looks as
fresh and vital as her new 56kg/8st
12lb figure makes her feel. Yellow
with lilac works surprisingly well,
but don't stop there. Try scarlet
with soft coral or dull biscuit
brown; try scarlet with sludgy
blues. Apple green with soft pale
blues, a stunning turquoise with
dull red, pinks, muted yellow or
oatmeal are other clever
combinations. You can add a splash
of colour with a t-shirt, beads,
bangles, ear-rings, belt, bag or
shoes.

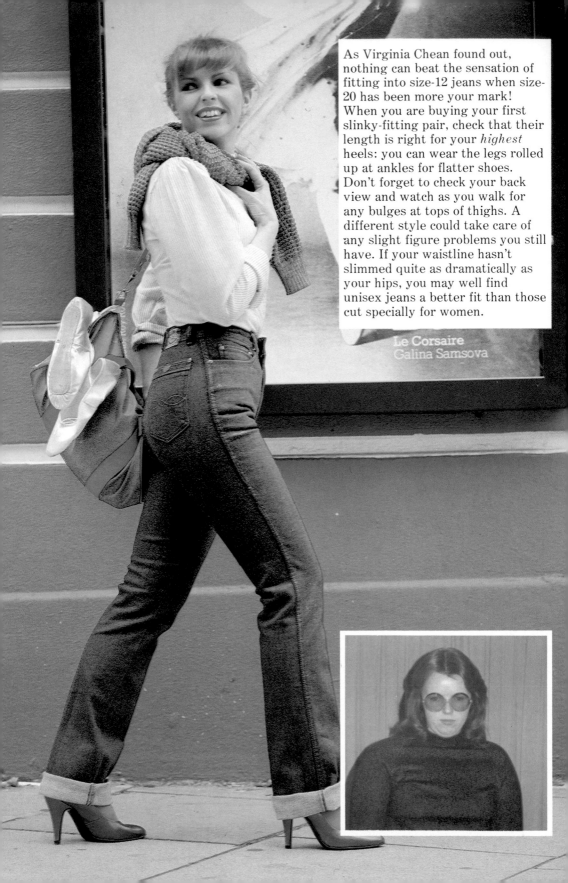

As Virginia Chean found out, nothing can beat the sensation of fitting into size-12 jeans when size-20 has been more your mark! When you are buying your first slinky-fitting pair, check that their length is right for your *highest* heels: you can wear the legs rolled up at ankles for flatter shoes. Don't forget to check your back view and watch as you walk for any bulges at tops of thighs. A different style could take care of any slight figure problems you still have. If your waistline hasn't slimmed quite as dramatically as your hips, you may well find unisex jeans a better fit than those cut specially for women.

Le Corsaire
Galina Samsova

a bowl with cheese and garlic salt. Add drained hot pasta and toss lightly until coated. Season and serve with green salad.

Snack 1 ☐ *150ml/¼ pint skimmed milk 20ml/2 rounded teaspoons drinking chocolate*   *4 ginger nuts or malted milk biscuits*

Snack 2 ☐ *1 can low-calorie soup, any flavour 1 crusty roll, brown or white*   *10ml/2 level teaspoons low-fat spread*

☐ If you completed the day without cheating at all, tick here and move on to Day 28.

☐ If you cheated, do a 'Saintly Day' tomorrow (page 253) instead of the set menu.

☐ If you do not eat one meal or snack that you are allowed, tick this box and save up for a 'Naughty Day'. When you have two ticks saved, you can do any of the Thoroughly Naughty Day's Menus *instead* of your next day's diet.

Exercise Day 27

MORNING ☐ Repeat Exercise 1: 5 times

☐ Repeat Exercise 2: 5 times to right
5 times to left

☐ Repeat Exercise 3: 5 times circling left and right with right foot
5 times circling left and right with left foot

☐ Repeat Exercise 4: touch the floor 15 times

☐ Repeat Exercise 5: bend to left and right 15 times

☐ Repeat Exercise 6: circle to left 15 times
circle to right 15 times

☐ Repeat Exercise 7: criss-cross 20 times

☐ Repeat Exercise 8: stretch 5 times

☐ Repeat Exercise 9: touch left foot and sit up
touch right foot and sit up 15 times

☐ Repeat Exercise 10: floor-walk to wall and back 5 times

☐ Repeat Exercise 11: arch spine and lower 3 times

☐ Repeat Exercise 12: raise left then right leg 15 times

LUNCHTIME ☐ Walk for 31 minutes, marking your position 11 minutes from your starting point. Turn and briskly walk to your marked position in 16 minutes, then jog the final stretch.

EVENING ☐ Run to the top of the stairs and down again 4 times. Jog for 10 minutes.

Or ☐ Jog for 20 minutes:
1st 5-minute jog
2nd 5-minute jog
3rd 5-minute jog
4th 5-minute jog

Then ☐ Run-skip 200 times.

Then ☐ Jump-skip 150 times.

☐ *Instead of your evening exercise, you could go to a swimming pool and spend half an hour steadily swimming. Sorry, paddling doesn't count. If you don't know how to swim this is a good time to decide to take lessons. Or you can go for a bicycle ride for at least 45 minutes.*

Bedtime Relaxer ☐

Are you still wearing the same colours you did 5 years ago? You could be tying yourself down to the same safe shades and missing out on a whole new spectrum of colour flattery. Perhaps consider shades a little brighter or softer? Take, for example, the vibrant primaries: blues, reds, yellows. Undiluted, they could well be too overpowering, but try them a shade up or down, plain or mixed. Next time you shop, try first of all the colours you would normally reject.

Brighten with ivory
Close to the face, ivory is kind. Or try a creamier tone, especially if your teeth are not very white and will look dingy by comparison. A crisp blouse, or a floppy bow in ivory or cream, will light up your face. Wear a creamy jacket with a light or darker skirt matched to shirt.

Today's special treatment
See the colour combinations used in our fashion transformations (between pages 240 1). Try the colour hints above and add to your colourscope. Try dyeing: practise on that old slip or shirt you planned to throw away. Use a cold water dye or one of those which can be tipped into the washing machine.

Cleanse, tone, moisturize
Cleanse, tone and moisturize your face in the morning and at night.

Hair livener
For dry hair only: massage scalp, see page 61, Day 7.

Skin spring clean
Repeat special treatment from page 22, Day 1.

Neck treat
Repeat treatment from page 49, Day 5.

Shopping Checklist Day 28

Choose your meals, then write in by each relevant item the amount you require.

Amount required		*Amount required*
Fruit and Vegetables		Low-fat natural
Carrots		yogurt
Celery		Low-fat spread
Lettuce		Skimmed milk
Mushrooms		**Grocery**
Onion		Bran breakfast cereal
Tomatoes		Brown rice
Apple		Crispbreads
Grapes		Crumpets
Melon		Low-calorie soup
Pear		Pineapple canned in
Frozen Foods		natural juice or
Oven or grill chips		low-calorie syrup
Peas		Raisins or sultanas
Meat, Poultry and Fish		Ribbon noodles
Minute steak		Wholemeal bread
Rump steak		**Store Cupboard**
Streaky bacon		Ground ginger
Dairy Produce/Eggs		Honey
Butter		Oil-free French
Cottage cheese		dressing
Curd cheese		Salt and pepper
Edam or Tendale		
cheese		
Eggs		

Diet Day 28

☐ *275ml/½ pint skimmed milk or reconstituted low-fat powdered milk*

BREAKFAST/SUPPER

Either ☐ *2 tomatoes, grilled without fat; 2 rashers streaky bacon, well grilled; 1 slice wholemeal bread, 40g/1½oz*

Or ☐ *1 egg, size 3, boiled; 1 small slice wholemeal bread, 25g/1oz; 5ml/1 level teaspoon low-fat spread*

Or ☐ *25g/1oz any bran breakfast cereal; 60ml/4 level tablespoons low-fat natural yogurt; 15ml/1 level tablespoon raisins or sultanas*

LIGHT MEAL

Either to eat at home
Soup, Crumpet plus Fruit

☐ 1 small can low calorie soup,   50g/2oz cottage cheese
   any flavour   1 medium apple or pear
1 crumpet
Start with soup. Toast crumpet on one side. Spread other side with cottage cheese and grill to heat through. Follow with fruit.

Or to take to work
Soup, Cottage Cheese plus Fruit

☐ 1 sachet instant low-calorie   4 crispbreads
   soup, any flavour   1 medium apple or pear
113g/4oz carton cottage
   cheese, any flavour except
   'with Cheddar'
Start with soup. Eat cottage cheese with crispbreads and follow with fruit.

MAIN MEAL

Either a quick recipe
Grilled Steak and Chips

☐ 115g/4oz minute steak   2 tomatoes
115g/4oz oven or grill chips
Grill minute steak on each side. Grill or bake chips as instructed on packet. Grill tomatoes and serve with steak and chips.

Or a keen cook's recipe **Ginger Melon plus Beef Stroganoff**

☐

250g/8oz slice melon
5ml/1 level teaspoon ground ginger (optional)
25g/1oz ribbon noodles, raw
75g/3oz rump steak
5ml/1 level teaspoon butter
½ small onion
50g/2oz button mushrooms
Salt and pepper
30ml/2 tablespoons low-fat natural yogurt
115g/4oz peas

Start with melon sprinkled with ginger. Boil noodles as instructed on packet. Remove fat from steak and cut meat into thin strips. Melt butter in a small pan and add chopped onion and mushrooms. Cook gently for 10 minutes. Add steak and seasoning and cook for a further 5-10 minutes. Carefully stir in the yogurt. Serve on the noodles with boiled peas.

Or if you prefer to eat vegetarian **Cheese Medley Salad**

☐

25g/1oz brown rice, raw
2 sticks celery
2 carrots
2 canned pineapple rings in natural juice or low-calorie syrup
50g/2oz grapes
30ml/2 tablespoons oil-free French dressing
Lettuce
40g/1½oz Edam or Tendale cheese
2 tomatoes

Cook rice in boiling salted water until just tender, about 30 minutes. Chop celery; grate carrots, drain and chop pineapple; halve grapes. Drain rice, rinse under cold water and drain again. Mix in a large bowl with celery, carrot, pineapple, grapes and dressing. Turn out onto a bed of lettuce. Surround with cubes of cheese and tomato wedges.

Snack 1

☐

2 small slices wholemeal bread, 25g/1oz each, toasted
10ml/2 level teaspoons low-fat spread
20ml/4 level teaspoons honey

Snack 2

☐

115g/4oz curd cheese
4 sticks celery
2 crispbreads

☐ If you completed the day without cheating at all, tick here and move on to Day 29.

☐ If you cheated, do a 'Saintly Day' tomorrow (page 253) instead of the set menu.

☐ If you do not eat one meal or snack that you are allowed, tick this box and save up for a 'Naughty Day'. When you have two ticks saved, you can do any of the Thoroughly Naughty Day's Menus *instead* of your next day's diet.

Exercise Day 28

MORNING ☐ Repeat Exercise 1: 5 times

☐ Repeat Exercise 2: 5 times to right
5 times to left

☐ Repeat Exercise 3: 5 times circling left and right with right foot
5 times circling left and right with left foot

☐ Repeat Exercise 4: touch the floor 15 times

☐ Repeat Exercise 5: bend to left and right 15 times

☐ Repeat Exercise 6: circle to left 15 times
circle to right 15 times

☐ Repeat Exercise 7: criss-cross 20 times

☐ Repeat Exercise 8: stretch 5 times

☐ Repeat Exercise 9: touch left foot and sit up
touch right foot and sit up 15 times

☐ Repeat Exercise 10: floor-walk to wall and back 5 times

☐ Repeat Exercise 11: arch spine and lower 3 times

☐ Repeat Exercise 12: raise left then right leg 15 times

Exercise 13 ☐ Stand up straight moving shoulders back, feet together and stretch the spine upwards. Feel yourself growing taller. Relax slightly and bring arms up so that fingers touch across chest and elbows are level with hands. Move arms out and back keeping them straight.

Clasp hands behind back and bend backwards from waist letting head fall back. Bend forward bringing hands, still clasped, up as far as possible. Try to relax neck muscles and hold forward position while counting to 5. Let go of hands and stand up straight.

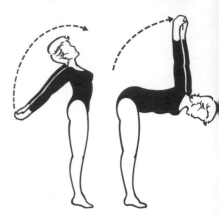

LUNCHTIME ☐ Walk for 32 minutes, marking your position 12 minutes from your starting point. Turn and briskly walk to your marked position in 16 minutes, then jog the final stretch.

EVENING ☐ Run to the top of the stairs and down again 4 times. Jog for 10 minutes.

Or ☐ Jog for 20 minutes:
1st 5-minute jog
2nd 5-minute jog
3rd 5-minute jog
4th 5-minute jog

Then ☐ Run-skip 200 times.

Then ☐ Jump-skip 200 times.

Bedtime Relaxer ☐

Beauty Day 28

Make this countdown day. Assess your progress. Check your body from head to toe.

Your hair
Oiliness should now be more under control. Restrict the scalp massage to once or twice a week, but massage shampoo in well when washing hair and rinse over and over

again. Dryness should be less of a problem. Continue massaging 2 to 3 times a week. Shampoo regularly. Signs that a shampoo is needed are increased oiliness, limp locks and irritating scalp.

Your skin
Silkier all over. Your face looking fresher? Keep the tingle treatment, page 22, Day 1, in reserve and use it fortnightly or monthly. Compensate dry skin by using body lotion regularly and especially guard against wear and tear on elbows, knees and ankles. Be kind to your neck and be lavish with moisturizer. Continue your daily cleanse, tone and moisturize routine for your face.

Your hands
Use hand lotion as a daily habit and continue your weekly manicure.

Your feet
Keep them comfortable. Reject shoes which pinch and take time to find shoes which are shaped to your foot. Give yourself a pedicure once a fortnight.

Today's special treatment
Check the following:

☐ * Back for blemishes. If spots are not fully cleared continue the spotty back treatment every other day.

☐ * Hair roots for regrowth if you have used a colorant. Make an appointment with your hairdresser or recolour yourself.

☐ * Anywhere you have used a depilatory. Check for re-growth; you'll need to do this every 2 days if hair is dark. Your props: a looking glass in daylight. Stroke fingertips over skin lightly to detect roughness.

☐ * Eyebrows for tweezering. These will need doing every 7-10 days.

Cleanse, tone, moisturize ☐ Cleanse, tone and moisturize your face in the morning and at night.

Elbows ☐ Still rough or discoloured? Mix lemon juice with a little salt and rub in. Rinse off after 5 to 10 minutes and apply body lotion.

Manicure ☐ Repeat manicure from page 54, Day 6.

Shopping Checklist Day 29

Choose your meals, then write in by each relevant item the amount you require.

Amount required	*Amount required*
Fruit and Vegetables	**Grocery**
Cabbage red or white	Bran breakfast cereal
Celery	Butter beans
Cucumber	Crispbreads
Green or red pepper	Dried apricots
Lettuce	Jam or fruit tart
Mushrooms	Peanuts
Onion	Pizza
Parsley	Raisins
Tomatoes	Salmon spread
Watercress	Walnut halves
Apples	Wholemeal bread
Bananas	**Store Cupboard**
Frozen Foods	Chopped parsley
Individual mousse	Dried mixed herbs
Pizza	Jam or marmalade
Meat, Poultry and Fish	Low-calorie salad
Streaky bacon	dressing
Dairy Produce/Eggs	Mustard
Cottage cheese	Nutmeg
Eggs	Oil-free French
Low-fat spread	dressing
Low-fat natural	Salt and pepper
yogurt	Tomato ketchup
Skimmed milk	

Diet Day 29

275ml/½ pint skimmed milk or reconstituted low-fat powdered milk

BREAKFAST/SUPPER MEAL

Either
2 eggs, size 3, scrambled with 15ml/1 tablespoon skimmed milk; 1 tomato, grilled without fat

Or
25g/1oz any bran breakfast cereal; 75ml/5 level tablespoons skimmed milk; 1 small banana, chopped

Or
2 small slices wholemeal bread, 25g/1oz each; 10ml/2 level teaspoons low-fat spread; 10ml/2 level teaspoons marmalade or jam

LIGHT MEAL

Either to eat at home
Mushroom and Bacon Toastie plus Banana

50g/2oz mushrooms   40g/1½oz
1 rasher streaky bacon   50g/2oz cottage cheese
1 slice wholemeal bread,   1 small banana
Slice mushrooms and poach in a little water. Cut bacon in half lengthways and grill well. Toast bread on one side. Put bacon, mushrooms and cottage cheese on untoasted side of bread and grill to heat through. Follow with banana.

Or to take to work
Salmon Crispbreads and Salad plus Fruit Tart

53g/1⅞oz pot salmon spread   25g/1oz mushrooms
2 crispbreads   15ml/1 tablespoon low-calorie
1 stick celery   salad dressing
¼ cucumber   1 small jam or fruit tart
Take pot of salmon spread to work separately and serve on crispbreads. Chop celery; dice cucumber and slice mushrooms. Put into a container and toss in salad dressing. Eat salad with crispbreads. Follow with jam or fruit tart.

Or if you prefer to eat vegetarian
Red Cabbage Crunch plus Banana

50g/2oz red or white cabbage   30ml/2 level tablespoons
3 sticks celery   low-fat natural yogurt
½ green pepper   15ml/1 tablespoon oil-free
1 green apple   French dressing
6 walnut halves   1 small banana
Shred cabbage and place in a bowl. Chop the celery and

235

green pepper then add to cabbage. Core and slice apple (dip in lemon juice if not eating immediately) and add to salad with walnuts, yogurt and oil-free French dressing. Toss to mix all ingredients. Follow with banana.

MAIN MEAL

Either a quick recipe **Pizza and Salad plus Mousse**

1 small pizza, about 115g/4oz
Lettuce
Cucumber
1 tomato

15ml/1 tablespoon oil-free French dressing
1 individual frozen mousse, any flavour

Cook pizza as instructed on packet. Serve with salad of lettuce, cucumber and tomato plus oil-free dressing. Follow with mousse.

Or a keen cook's recipe **Butter Bean Quiche plus Apricot and Apple Dessert**

25g/1oz onion
¼ red or green pepper
213g/7½oz can butter beans, drained
1 egg, size 3
75ml/5 level tablespoons low-fat natural yogurt
2.5ml/½ level teaspoon mustard
1.25ml/¼ level teaspoon dried mixed herbs
Salt and pepper

5ml/1 level teaspoon chopped parsley
45ml/3 level tablespoons fresh wholemeal breadcrumbs
Lettuce
Cucumber
Watercress
25g/1oz dried apricots
1 medium apple
Nutmeg

Chop onion and simmer in a little water for 3 minutes. Discard pith and seeds from pepper and dice flesh. Add to onion and cook for 2 minutes. Drain and place in an ovenproof dish with beans. Lightly beat egg and yogurt together; add mustard, herbs and seasoning. Pour over vegetables; sprinkle with parsley and breadcrumbs. Stand dish in a tin containing ½-inch water. Cook at 180°C/350°F, gas mark 4, for 25 minutes. Serve with green salad made from lettuce cucumber and watercress. Soak apricots in hot water for at least 2 hours. Save 15ml/1 tablespoon of the liquid and put it into a saucepan with apricots and peeled, cored and sliced apple. Sprinkle with a little nutmeg and cook very gently until the apple is tender.

Snack 1

30ml/2 level tablespoons raisins

15ml/1 level tablespoon peanuts

236

Snack 2 ☐ *2 rashers streaky bacon, well grilled*
15ml/1 tablespoon tomato ketchup

2 small slices wholemeal bread, 25g/1oz each

☐ If you completed the day without cheating at all, tick here and move on to Day 30.

☐ If you cheated, do a 'Saintly Day' tomorrow (page 253) instead of the set menu.

☐ If you do not eat one meal or snack that you are allowed, tick this box and save up for a 'Naughty Day'. When you have two ticks saved, you can do any of the Thoroughly Naughty Day's Menus *instead* of your next day's diet.

Exercise Day 29

MORNING ☐ Repeat Exercise 1: 5 times

☐ Repeat Exercise 2: 5 times to right
5 times to left

☐ Repeat Exercise 3: 5 times circling left and right with right foot
5 times circling left and right with left foot

☐ Repeat Exercise 4: touch the floor 15 times

☐ Repeat Exercise 5: bend to left and right 15 times

☐ Repeat Exercise 6: circle to left 15 times
circle to right 15 times

☐ Repeat Exercise 7: criss-cross 20 times

☐ Repeat Exercise 8: stretch 5 times

☐ Repeat Exercise 9: touch left foot and sit up
touch right foot and sit up 15 times

☐ Repeat Exercise 10: floor-walk to wall and back 5 times

☐ Repeat Exercise 11: arch spine and lower 3 times

☐ Repeat Exercise 12: raise left then right leg 15 times

☐ Repeat Exercise 13: do complete movement twice

LUNCHTIME ☐ Walk for 33 minutes, marking your position 13 minutes from your starting point. Turn and briskly walk to your marked position in 16 minutes, then jog the final stretch.

EVENING ☐ Run to the top of the stairs and down again 4 times. Jog for 10 minutes.

Or ☐ Jog for 20 minutes:
1st 5-minute jog
2nd 5-minute jog
3rd 5-minute jog
4th 5-minute jog

Then ☐ Run-skip 200 times.

Then ☐ Jump-skip 200 times.

Then ☐ Skip backwards 50 times. Circle rope backwards and jump up and down with your feet together. Keep your arms as high as possible as this helps to firm arm muscles.

Bedtime Relaxer ☐

Beauty Day 29

The biggest single thing that most women can do to take off years is to take off excess weight. But what else can make a terrific difference, too? Here are 10 artful ways to look years younger.

1. Think thin about make-up
Thick make-up lodges in any lines and wrinkles and emphasizes them. Use the thinnest possible layer of moisturizer, foundation and powder. Aim at a natural-looking glow of well-being — a slightly tanned effect can

help a lot, provided you use blusher to beat any sallowness.

2. Cheat away that chin
Posture can make all the difference: a head held high
instantly diminishes a heavy chin. Shading tricks rarely
work in daylight, and a camouflaged area can attract
attention because of its apparent grubbiness. But in
artificial light, lose years by being bolder; a brown blusher
or shader gently stroked on a double chin can play it down
effectively.

3. Pick a young hair colour
First rule for youthful flattery: tint any shade of greying
brown two tones lighter than the original colour; this is far
kinder to the complexion than going darker. Rule 2: young
hair isn't all one colour, so never have too dense a dye —
solid black is especially ageing. Rule 3: be careful that
bleached hair doesn't take on a yellow tinge; this can kill
any older complexion. Gentle ashy shades, if not over-pale,
give a face a far younger frame.

4. Get a swinging skirt
A young look is easy-going, full of movement, the reverse of
stiff and static. So get a skirt that swings — and stride out
to make it move. No fullness from the waist, please, if
heavyish hips loom below; an A-line is usually the kindest
cut.

5. Mascara lower lashes
If you offer no distraction in the area, under-eye crepiness
is more likely to show. So use mascara neatly and discreetly
on both upper *and* lower lashes, and switch the shade from
hard black to navy blue. This can make an attractively
youthful difference.

6. Boot out stodgy shoes
Whatever your leg shape, plain courts are the most
flattering style of all. Straps, especially the ankle kind, have
a foreshortening and fattening effect.

7. Avoid unflattering fabrics
Fabrics that are glittery, shaggy, furry, cheap-velvety or
bold-patterned, especially in Crimplene, all tend to add
inches — and *they* mean years.

8. Switch to support tights
Today's support tights can be so sheer that there's not the

slightest 'surgical' air about them. Many a model girl has them in her kit to fight leg fatigue. They can give the legs a long, firm line and youthful smoothness, especially in the calf and knee area. For maximum benefit, smooth them on first thing, *before* your legs have taken your body weight.

9. Take the 'up' options
A woman's basic beauty battle is against gravity, the force that would like to get everything about you drooping down. You fight it most efficiently by taking all possible 'up' options. Stud earrings rather than heavy pendants, for instance. Hair with top and side fullness instead of long dangly strands. A casual curly cut, with life and bounce, is very young-making — as long as it's not so short that it unkindly exposes the neck and jaw. Whatever your style, aim at a graceful frame for your face.

10. Look alive!
Youth is enthusiasm, vivacity, involvement — and dignity doesn't mean deadpan. Don't let it *all* hang out (miserable moments are best kept private) but cultivate the habit of letting every 'up' emotion show in your face. Smile . . .

Today's special treatment
Try out some of the tricks above and make this a 'feel good' day. Greet neighbours or colleagues with a sunny smile when you say 'Good day'. Pay a few compliments: sincerely making others feel good can give you a glow, too. Vow that, whatever the provocation, you're not going to let anyone upset you or make you angry for this 24 hours.

Cleanse, tone, moisturize
Cleanse, tone and moisturize your skin in the morning and at night.

Spotty back?
Soak in warm bath; scrub back with medicated soap, dry and dab with diluted antiseptic. Dust with medicated talc.

Pedicure
Repeat the pedicure from page 81, Day 9.

Shopping Checklist Day 30

Choose your meals, then write in by each relevant item the amount you require.

Amount required	*Amount required*
Fruit and Vegetables	Low-fat spread
Apple or pear	Skimmed milk
Carrots	**Grocery**
Celery	Bran breakfast cereal
Lettuce	Canned tomatoes
Mushrooms	Cream crackers
Onion	Raisins or sultanas
Red or green pepper	Wholemeal bread
Tomatoes	Wholewheat pasta
Frozen Foods	Wholewheat spaghetti
Choc-ice	**Store Cupboard**
Fish fingers	Garlic salt and
Mixed vegetables	black pepper
Oven or grill chips	Low-calorie salad
Peas	dressing
Meat, Poultry and Fish	Oregano or
Streaky bacon	mixed herbs
Dairy Produce/Eggs	Salt and pepper
Butter or margarine	
Cheddar,	
Double Gloucester	
or Stilton cheese	
Cottage cheese with	
pineapple	
Eggs	
Low-fat fruit yogurt	

Diet Day 30

☐ 275ml/½ pint skimmed milk or reconstituted low-fat powdered milk

BREAKFAST/SUPPER MEAL

Either ☐ 1 slice wholemeal bread, 40g/1½oz; 1 egg, size 3; 5ml/1 level teaspoon low-fat spread
Dip bread into beaten egg and fry in a non-stick pan greased with low-fat spread.

Or ☐ 25g/1oz any bran breakfast cereal; 75ml/5 level tablespoons skimmed milk; 30ml/2 level tablespoons raisins or sultanas

Or ☐ 2 rashers streaky bacon, well grilled; 2 tomatoes, grilled without fat; 1 small slice wholemeal bread, 25g/1oz

LIGHT MEAL

Either to eat at home
Carrot, Cheese and Raisin Salad plus Apple
☐ 115g/4oz carrots   1 small carton cottage cheese
25g/1oz raisins   with pineapple
                                    Lettuce
Grate carrot and mix with raisins and cottage cheese. Shred as much lettuce as you wish and put onto a serving dish. Top with cheese and carrot mixture. Follow with apple.

Or to take to work
Pasta and Vegetable Medley plus Fruit
☐ 25g/1oz wholewheat pasta   15ml/1 level tablespoon low-
150g/5oz frozen mixed   calorie salad dressing
   vegetables   1 medium apple or pear
¼ red pepper
Cook pasta in boiling salted water. Rinse in cold water and drain. Cook frozen mixed vegetables as directed on packet. Rinse in cold water and drain. Chop red pepper and mix all ingredients together. Take to work in a container. Follow with apple or pear.

MAIN MEAL

Either a quick recipe
Fish Fingers and Chips
☐ 4 fish fingers   115g/4oz oven or grill chips
115g/4oz peas
Grill fish fingers without fat. Boil peas and cook oven or grill chips as instructed. Serve fish fingers with peas and chips.

Or a keen
cook's recipe
**Spaghetti with
Mushroom Sauce**

☐

50g/2oz wholewheat
   spaghetti
1 small onion
5ml/1 level teaspoon butter
   or margarine
¼ red or green pepper
1 stick celery

50g/2oz mushrooms
227g/8oz can tomatoes
Pinch oregano or mixed
   herbs
Garlic salt and black pepper
1 small fruit yogurt,
   any flavour

Boil spaghetti as instructed on packet. Chop onion; fry in
butter in a small saucepan until soft. Discard white pith and
seeds from pepper; cut flesh into strips. Add to pan with
chopped celery. Fry gently for 2-3 minutes; add sliced
mushrooms, tomatoes and oregano; season and cover.
Simmer for 10 minutes. Add a little water if the sauce
seems to be sticking. Serve sauce on boiled spaghetti.
Follow with fruit yogurt.

Snack 1 ☐   *1 individual choc-ice*

Snack 2 ☐

25g/1oz Cheddar, Double
   Gloucester or Stilton
   cheese

2 cream crackers
1 medium apple

Exercise Day 30

MORNING ☐   Repeat Exercise 1: 5 times

☐   Repeat Exercise 2: 5 times to right
5 times to left

☐   Repeat Exercise 3: 5 times circling left and right with
right foot
5 times circling left and right with left foot

☐   Repeat Exercise 4: touch the floor 15 times

☐   Repeat Exercise 5: bend to left and right 15 times

☐   Repeat Exercise 6: circle to left 15 times
circle to right 15 times

☐ Repeat Exercise 7: criss-cross 20 times

☐ Repeat Exercise 8: stretch 5 times

☐ Repeat Exercise 9: touch left foot and sit up
touch right foot and sit up 15 times

☐ Repeat Exercise 10: floor-walk to wall and back 5 times

☐ Repeat Exercise 11: arch spine and lower 3 times

☐ Repeat Exercise 12: raise left then right leg 15 times

☐ Repeat Exercise 13: do complete movement 3 times

LUNCHTIME ☐ Walk for 35 minutes, marking your position 15 minutes
from your starting point. Turn and briskly walk to your
marked position in 16 minutes, then jog the final stretch.

EVENING ☐ Run to the top of the stairs and down again 4 times. Jog
for 10 minutes.

Or ☐ Jog for 20 minutes:
1st 5-minute jog
2nd 5-minute jog
3rd 5-minute jog
4th 5-minute jog

Then ☐ Run-skip 200 times.

Then ☐ Jump-skip 200 times.

Then ☐ Skip backwards 100 times.

Bedtime Relaxer ☐

☐ This now completes your 30-day exercise plan. Keep on
repeating your exercises every day and it will help you to
keep in shape. If you still have particular problem areas,
such as your thighs or stomach, start to work in an exercise
every day specifically to help. Here are some excellent
problem area trimmers:

**Special exercise
to thin thighs** Kneel on a carpet with your
knees slightly apart and lean
backwards, keeping your
upper body rounded
forwards.

245

Without moving your upper body, try to thrust your pelvis forward from your hips and push forwards until your thighs are upright.

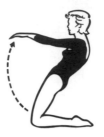

Follow through with your upper body, lift your arms and bring your body upright. Aim to get your pelvis and thighs completely forward first before you move your upper body — that's the part of you that must do the work. The lower you manage to go back initially, the greater the pull on those reluctant thigh muscles. You will feel them working really hard.

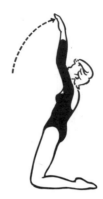

Special exercise to flatten your stomach

Lie on the floor with your legs raised and slightly bent at the knees and your arms outstretched.

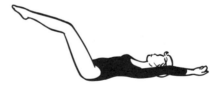

Tilt your pelvis and raise the upper part of your body and hold onto your legs.

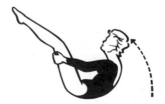

Then let go and raise your arms as far back as you can above your head. Keep your legs in the air and hold. You'll feel unpleasant pulls in your stomach but try and count up to 10. Lower your arms and legs, have a rest and start again.

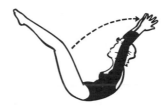

Special exercises to trim your waist Do extra sessions of exercises 5 and 6 which are very good waist-willowers.

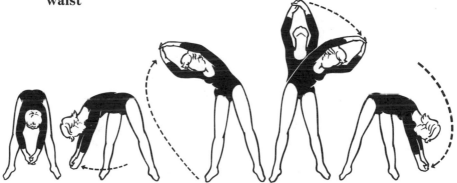

Beauty Day 30

If you know you are looking good, doesn't it make a difference to your day? Able to cope and confident, you help to make nice things happen — instead of shrinking back and letting every niggle bring you down. Psychologists call it 'positive reflex': a firm-minded refusal to take a downbeat point of view. The aim of this book has been to show you how to become slim and shapely, how to capitalize on your most attractive features. Don't let it all end here!

Do something new
Swimming, tennis, badminton, a keep-fit class. Any of these
will help keep you in shape, introduce you to new friends.
Ask at the Citizens Advice Bureau and your local library
about social/hobby/help groups. They should have a list of
these on file (and they may include your local *Slimming
Magazine* Club). Or alternatively you could ring your local
authority's recreation or leisure section.

Keep Active
The more active you are, the less likely you are to put back
any lost pounds. Here are the activities which will burn up
the most calories:
Badminton: playing with average effort
Basketball: lots of very fast running and jumping
Circuit training: climbing gymnasium bars and other
equipment
Cycling: the faster you peddle the better
Dancing: disco and country better than ballroom
Gardening: particularly digging
Hockey: playing a reasonably vigorous game
Horse riding: trotting or galloping
Ice-skating: at an average pace
Jogging: at a comfortable steady pace
Netball: playing a reasonably fast game
Rowing: pulling quite hard
Skipping: one of the best calorie burners of all
Squash: a very strenuous sport if played hard
Swimming: an ideal exercise since it uses all the muscles
Tennis: the harder the game the better
Walking: fast and particularly uphill

Widen your horizons
Take a real interest in the things which interest other
people. You'll learn a lot, boost your stock of small talk, and
find a lot more friendliness.

Shrug it off
Yesterday may have been a disaster, or even the whole of
last week. But yesterday is just history. Learn any lessons
it can teach you, then bid it a firm goodbye. Think carefully
about all aspects of a problem — it's easier that way to
decide on a clear-headed solution. Remember: if it's a
problem, there's a solution. If there *isn't* a solution, then it's
a fact of life — and you'll feel a lot better if you decide
today that you're going to live with it with a good grace and
a sense of humour.

Increase your self-confidence!

Have you always thought of yourself as a rather shy person, not at all comfortable about encountering new people? Has a surplus weight problem tended to sap your social self-confidence? Well, now *that* problem is well on the wane let's have a look at any remaining miseries you may find in meeting people. And we promise — confidently! — that what follows will really help you . . .

When you cringe at the idea of some encounter, you need to look really hard at what lies behind your reaction. For a start, pinpoint which people tend to make you particularly nervous: younger, older, thinner? Then look at the situations that usually trigger off your tensions. Does having to make small talk scare you? Is a crowd more frightening than just two or three people? Etc., etc. The aim of all the detective work is this: nailing the precise cause of any fear — putting it into plain, honest words, preferably out loud — usually puts the problem into perspective, and reduces the panic. And once you've stopped it being blind panic, you can begin to consider the counter-measures most likely to yield a cure. Let's look at what a truth-session might turn up . . .

'I'm sure they won't like me.'
Yes, you can safely assume some people won't like you. Big deal! No one ever appeals to everybody: for proof, just consider some of the life partners that people you know have picked! So it makes sense not to overload meetings with exaggerated expectations, nice or nasty. If you always go along to any gathering prepared to take an interest and meet anyone politely halfway, you'll find your share of pleasant, responsive people. Just don't expect soul-to-soul meetings every time; we all need a broad mix of relationships at varying levels of intimacy. Sometimes it will be your day; sometimes it won't. Simply resolve to meet both sorts with a smile and in a philosophical frame of mind. That, in any case, is infinitely more appealing than a glowering take-me-as-I-am defiance or a poor-little-worthless-me approach. The self-absorption implicit in both these attitudes does not leave much interest to spare for others — and there are few surer social turn-offs than that.

'They are all nicer-looking/thinner/more intelligent/better off/better educated/more worthwhile than I am.'
The short answer to this kind of 'inner' dialogue is: 'So

what?' Even if there were some agreed scale to measure and compare all personal qualities (there isn't and never can be), we would all find plenty of people 'above' and vast armies 'below'.

This sort of ratings game is juvenile; adults accept that we are all different. Everyone has a unique worth, with no need for any 'pardon me for living' apology.

It's sensible, of course, to aim to improve anything — from the width of one's seat to the breadth of one's knowledge — that is sapping self-confidence. There are so many things that can be changed for the better; so why be lumbered with them? Meanwhile, however, realize that you already have plenty of things in your favour as you are: a warm smile and an optimistic outlook are particularly worth parading. Accept that everybody has good points and bad. If you decide from now on to concentrate socially only on the good ones, in yourself and in others, it makes everyday encounters much more relaxed and enjoyable.

'I'm so bad at meeting people, I wonder why I bother.'
You keep on bothering because it's a sound, healthy human instinct to stay in touch with the people you know and to give yourself the chance of forming fresh relationships. And, by now, you should be beginning to see how you can bother to better purpose. There are old ideas you can re-examine, new skills you can learn to make encounters much less of a strain . . . But what if somebody won't bother to bring her social fears out into the open and take positive steps to combat them? Then a likely answer is that, however odd it seems, it suits her to stay obviously awkward and unsure. Being able to moan to a friend: 'Why did you insist on taking me along? I told you no one would like me' can confirm old feelings of low self-esteem and is a fine excuse for making no further effort. Strangely, too, there's a cosy comfort in familiar feelings, even uncomfortable ones like rejection. And the person who displays herself as unsure and ill at ease is subconsciously sending out the social message: 'Look, I'm no threat, no competition to you; so why not give me an easier time?'

What do you do once you've thought hard about these internal reactions? The next step is to consider how they affect your outward behaviour. One of the most destructive ideas many of us carry through from childhood is the concept that other people somehow must know how we really feel inside. They don't, alas. They can't be sure unless we actually come out with our feelings; all they can do otherwise is judge by our outward behaviour. So check that yours isn't giving a false impression; for instance, shyness coming over as standoffishness . . .

Social 'nerves' show in other ways. People go blotchy; they blush; they um-and-er, go silent or giggle. Making yourself aware of what happens in your case means you can see if any symptoms can be controlled. You can usually take useful steps if you've a mind to. A woman whose 'nerves' always expressed themselves in blotchy red patches on her upper chest and neck, finally accepted that this would happen and took to wearing pretty but high-necked clothes on social occasions. And, because she then relaxed about them, the blotches stopped.

The best thing you can do in advance of any stressful situation is as much 'homework' as possible — find out the precise nature of the occasion, what people usually wear, etc. — but then make up your mind to be philosophical. The person others automatically warm to is someone who is on good terms with herself: she's tolerant of her own shortcomings as well as other people's and she does not take herself too seriously. People instinctively tend to shy away from someone who looks like being a burden. That is why looking nervous and unsure has such a negative effect. So aim to appear cheerful even if you don't feel it; very often the pretence becomes reality sooner than you had dared to hope. Being busy often helps: can you hand some food round, for example? A hostess often welcomes aid. Be brave enough to say: 'Do let me take round those sausage rolls — it helps me to get over being shy.' Then she'll know how you feel and may let you help even if she doesn't need it. It's all part of the admitting-your-needs campaign!

Other practical ploys apply. You'll only emphasize feelings of isolation if you cling uneasily to the edge of a crowd who know each other well. Better to seek out another shy soul . . . Beginnings are important. If they don't come easily, take time to work out a few openings in advance. The 'Have you noticed?' sort can work well. 'Have you noticed far fewer people are smoking lately?' Or: 'On my way here, I was thinking isn't it odd that . . .' All questions that can't be easily dismissed with a straight yes or no . . . Sometimes, shy people get desperate because they can't see how to end an encounter gracefully. Useful getaway gambits include: 'Excuse me, but I promised to telephone my aunt/the baby sitter/my father before 8 p.m.' Or: 'Ah, there's So-and-So. I've been meaning to snatch a private word with her for ages. Do, please, excuse me.' Or (and we like this one's basic honesty): 'It doesn't show too much, I hope, but I've always been shy, so I've made this resolution to talk to at least 4 people this evening. I'll certainly be lucky if they're all as nice as you.'

The whole secret of coping with the misery of meeting people — any situation that you dread — is to sort out very clearly in your own mind what it really is that causes these feelings of panic. Invariably it will be something from the past which may have mattered once but should not be hindering your happiness now. Swap such limp little girl thoughts as: 'They won't like me' for a grown-up: 'More fool them!'

The truth is that probably half the people who look relaxed and confident at any gathering have fought or are fighting the same fears which are afflicting you. If you really want to you can take the hell out of hello.

Saintly Day Menus

If you had a bad day and didn't manage to stick to your diet, you must follow a Saintly Day Menu immediately to repair the damage. You can choose any breakfast from the list below and two of the following light meals. That is all you are allowed for the day except black tea or coffee (with artificial sweetener only), water, low-calorie mixer drinks or squashes and yeast extract drinks. These you can drink in unlimited quantities. You are not allowed any milk except where it is mentioned in a meal.

BREAKFASTS

Choose any one of these a day

Toast and Marmalade	*2 slices wholemeal bread, 25g/1oz each 10ml/2 level teaspoons low-fat spread*	*10ml/2 level teaspoons marmalade or jam*
Fruit Juice plus Cereal	*115ml/4floz unsweetened orange juice*	*25g/1oz cereal, any brand 115ml/4floz skimmed milk*
Muesli Yogurt	*25g/1oz muesli 1 small carton natural yogurt*	*25g/1oz black grapes*
Grapefruit Boiled Egg	*½ grapefruit 1 egg, size 3, boiled 1 small slice bread, 25g/1oz*	*5ml/1 level teaspoon low-fat spread*
Bacon and Tomatoes	*2 rashers streaky bacon, well grilled 2 tomatoes, grilled*	*1 small slice wholemeal bread, 25g/1oz, toasted*

253

Choose any two of these each day

Cod in Sauce and Vegetables *1 pack frozen cod in cheese sauce*   *150g/5oz mixed vegetables, frozen*

Cook the fish as directed on packet. Serve with boiled mixed vegetables.

Ham Steak with Pineapple and Sweetcorn *1 ham or bacon steak (100g/3½oz raw)*   *115g/4oz sweetcorn, frozen or canned*
1 ring pineapple, canned in natural juice, drained

Grill ham or bacon steak and heat pineapple under the grill. Serve with boiled sweetcorn.

Roast Beef with Salad *75g/3oz lean roast topside of beef*   *1 tomato*
142g/5oz carton coleslaw in low-calorie dressing

Discard all visible fat from the beef. Serve the lean with coleslaw and tomato.

Grilled Liver with Mushrooms and Tomato *115g/4oz lamb's or pig's liver*   *1 tomato*
115g/4oz mushrooms

Grill the liver and tomato without added fat. Serve with mushrooms, poached in a little stock or water.

Sausages with Baked Beans and Tomatoes *2 beef chipolata sausages*   *150g/5.3oz can baked beans in tomato sauce*
2 tomatoes

Grill the sausages and tomatoes without added fat. Serve with the heated baked beans.

Fish Fingers with Peas *3 fish fingers*   *15ml/1 tablespoon tomato ketchup*
115g/4oz peas, frozen

Grill the fish fingers without added fat. Serve with boiled peas and tomato ketchup.

Grilled Chicken with Vegetables *1 chicken breast, 175g/6oz*   *150g/5oz cauliflower, fresh or frozen*
115g/4oz peas, frozen

Grill the chicken breast and discard the skin. Serve chicken with boiled peas and cauliflower.

Kidneys with Spaghetti

2 lamb's kidneys

213g/7½oz can spaghetti rings with tomato sauce

Grill the kidneys without added fat and serve with the hot spaghetti.

Cod in Butter Sauce with Broccoli

1 packet frozen cod in butter sauce

115g/4oz broccoli, fresh or frozen

Cook the cod in butter sauce as directed on the packet. Serve with the boiled broccoli.

Roast Pork

75g/3oz roast leg of pork
15ml/1 level tablespoon unsweetened apple sauce
30ml/2 tablespoons thin, fat-free gravy

115g/4oz Brussels sprouts, fresh or frozen
115g/4oz carrots, fresh or frozen

Discard all visible fat and crackling from pork. Serve with apple sauce, gravy and boiled vegetables.

Cottage Cheese and Egg Salad

113g/4oz carton cottage cheese with chives
1 egg, size 3
2 tomatoes

Unlimited lettuce, cucumber, cress, onion and green pepper
15ml/1 tablespoon oil-free French dressing

Hard boil the egg. Cool and shell and serve with cottage cheese and salad vegetables (sprinkled with oil-free French dressing).

Roast Beef and Vegetables

100g/3½oz packet frozen sliced roast beef in gravy
15ml/1 level tablespoon horseradish sauce

50ml/2 level tablespoons instant mashed potato powder
115g/4oz carrots

Cook beef and make up potato as instructed on the packet. Serve beef with potato, horseradish sauce and boiled carrots.

Fish Cakes with Baked Beans

2 fish cakes

150g/5.3oz can baked beans in tomato sauce

Grill fish cakes without added fat. Serve with hot beans.

Curd Cheese and Cucumber Roll

1 crusty bread roll
50g/2oz curd cheese

Few slices cucumber

Split the roll and fill with curd cheese and cucumber.

Chicken Sandwich   *2 small slices bread*   *25g/1oz cooked chicken*
                        (25g/1oz each)   *Mustard and cress*
                      15g/½oz low-fat spread

Scrape the bread with low-fat spread. Discard any skin from chicken, then make into a sandwich with the bread and mustard and cress.

Cheese and Ham Sandwich   *2 small slices bread, 25g/1oz*   *15ml/1 level tablespoon*
                        each   *cheese spread*
                                           25g/1oz lean cooked ham

Spread bread with cheese. Discard all visible fat from ham and make into a sandwich with bread.

Prawn Salad   *115g/4oz prawns*   *15ml/1 tablespoon oil-free*
                  30ml/2 tablespoons low-   *French dressing*
                    calorie seafood sauce   *2 crispbreads*
                  2 tomatoes
                  Lettuce, watercress,
                    cucumber, celery, green
                    pepper

Mix prawns with seafood sauce. Quarter the tomatoes. Make a green salad with a selection of the vegetables and toss in oil-free French dressing. Arrange the prawns, tomatoes and green salad on a plate and serve with crispbreads.

Shepherd's Pie and Green Beans   *1 frozen shepherd's pie*
                        115g/4oz French beans or
                        haricots vert, fresh or
                        frozen

Cook the shepherd's pie as instructed on the packet. Serve with boiled beans.

Roast Lamb   *75g/3oz roast leg of lamb*   *115g/4oz runner beans, fresh*
                15ml/1 tablespoon mint sauce   *or frozen*
                115g/4oz cabbage, fresh or
                  frozen

Discard all visible fat from the lamb. Serve lean with mint sauce and boiled vegetables.

Grilled Plaice with Mixed Vegetables

150g/5oz plaice fillet
7g/¼oz low-fat spread
115g/4oz mixed vegetables, frozen

15ml/1 tablespoon tomato ketchup

Dot the plaice with low-fat spread and grill. Serve with boiled vegetables and tomato ketchup.

Baked Beans on Toast

225g/7.9oz can baked beans with tomato sauce

1 small slice bread, 25g/1oz

Heat the beans and serve on toasted bread.

Chicken Drumsticks with Stir Fry Vegetables

2 chicken drumsticks
115g/4oz Bird's Eye Stir Fry Continental or Country Style Vegetables

7g/¼oz butter
2.5ml/½ teaspoon oil

Grill the drumsticks and discard skin. Cook vegetables in butter and oil as instructed on the packet and serve with chicken drumsticks.

Smoked Haddock and Peas

1 packet frozen buttered Scottish smoked haddock, 170g/6oz

115g/4oz peas, frozen

Cook the smoked haddock as instructed on the packet and serve with boiled peas.

Thoroughly Naughty Day Menus

When you have saved up two ticks on any of your 30-Day Menus, you can treat yourself to a 'naughty' day. Use this section if you are eating out — we have given five restaurant choices. Or use these menus to give yourself a little treat if you are feeling particularly low or bored. Some slimmers feel that, psychologically, they need to 'break out' occasionally on a diet and if you use these menus you can do that without slowing your weight loss.

MAIN MEAL AT A STEAK BAR

Milk allowance *275ml/½ pint skimmed milk to use in tea and coffee*

Breakfast *1 egg, size 3* *5ml/1 level teaspoon low-fat*
1 crispbread *spread*
Boil the egg. Serve with the crispbread and low-fat spread.

Light Meal *113g/4oz cottage cheese, any* *2 crispbreads*
flavour except 'with *Cucumber*
Cheddar' *1 medium apple or pear*
Top the crispbreads with cottage cheese and sliced cucumber. Follow with the fruit.

Main meal at *Melon* *Salad (no dressing)*
a steak bar *225g/8oz steak, medium or* *Mustard*
well grilled (cut off any *Ice cream*
excess fat before eating) *Coffee with milk (ask for*
Garnish of tomato and *milk instead of cream if*
mushroom *it is not offered). 2 glasses*
Jacket baked potato, without *of wine, red or white*
butter or soured cream

MAIN MEAL AT A PIZZA HOUSE

Milk allowance *275ml/½ pint skimmed milk, extra to allowance*

258

Breakfast 25g/1oz any bran breakfast cereal
1 small banana

90ml/6 tablespoons skimmed milk, extra to allowance

Light Meal 1 crusty bread roll
15g/½oz low-fat spread
25g/1oz lean cooked ham

1 tomato
1 medium pear or peach or nectarine

Split the roll and spread with low-fat spread. Discard any visible fat from ham, then place in roll with sliced tomato. Follow with fruit.

Main meal from a pizza house 1 average pizza from a pizza house

1 cup coffee with milk
2 glasses wine, white or red

MAIN MEAL AT A HAMBURGER BAR

Milk allowance 275ml/½ pint skimmed milk for use in tea or coffee

Breakfast 1 slice wholemeal bread, 40g/1½oz
5ml/1 level teaspoon low-fat spread

10ml/1 rounded teaspoon marmalade or jam

Light meal 50g/2oz white cabbage
1 medium carrot
1 spring onion
1 stick celery
50g/2oz Edam or Tendale cheese

15ml/1 level tablespoon raisins or sultanas
45ml/3 level tablespoons natural low-fat yogurt
Salt and pepper

Shred cabbage; grate carrot; chop spring onion and celery. Cut cheese into small cubes. Mix all the ingredients together and season with salt and pepper.

Main meal (from a McDonalds) 1 Big Mac
1 small portion of French Fries

1 McDonald's Milk Shake, any flavour

MAIN MEAL FROM A CHINESE RESTAURANT

Milk allowance 275ml/½ pint skimmed milk to use in drinks

Breakfast   *25g/1oz any bran breakfast*   *75ml/5 tablespoons skimmed*
                  cereal   *milk, extra to allowance*

Light meal   *100g/3½oz can tuna in brine*   *30ml/2 tablespoons low-*
                  2 sticks celery   *calorie salad dressing*
                  1 small apple   *A squeeze of lemon juice*
                  Piece of cucumber,
                     approximately 5cm/2
                     inches

Drain and flake tuna. Slice celery. Core and dice apple. Dice cucumber. Toss apple in the lemon juice, then mix with all the other ingredients.

                  (For when you are eating as part of a group with a selection
                  of dishes)
Either   *4 large prawn crackers*   *1 Spring Roll*
Chinese meal 1 *60ml/4 tablespoons Chicken*   *2 Barbecued Spare Ribs*
                     and Mushrooms   *1 portion lychees*
                  60ml/4 tablespoons Prawn   *China tea*
                     Chop Suey
                  60ml/4 tablespoons fried
                     rice

Or   (If you are ordering your own dishes)
Chinese Meal 2 *1 portion Prawn Chop Suey*   *1 portion lychees*
                  1 portion Chicken Chow Mein   *China tea*
                  1 portion plain boiled rice

Or   (From a Take-Away)
Chinese Meal 3 *1 portion Beef in Oyster*   *1 portion fried rice*
                     Sauce   *1 portion lychees*

Or   (From a Take-Away)
Chinese Meal 4 *1 portion Barbecued Spare*   *1 portion plain boiled rice*
                     Ribs   *1 Spring Roll*

A CHIP-LOVER'S DAY

Milk allowance   *275ml/½ pint skimmed milk for use in tea or coffee*

Breakfast   *2 rashers streaky bacon,*   *150g/5.3oz can baked beans*
well grilled   *with tomato sauce*

Light meal   *1 tomato*   *15ml/1 tablespoon low-calorie*
Lettuce, cucumber, mustard   *salad dressing*
and cress, spring onions   *1 medium pear, peach or*
75g/3oz corned beef   *nectarine*
Make a salad with the vegetables and serve with the corned beef and dressing. Follow with the fruit.

Main meal   *175g/6oz grill chips or oven*   *15ml/1 tablespoon brown*
chips   *sauce or tomato ketchup*
2 eggs, size 3   *1 medium banana*
Oil
Cook chips as instructed on the packet. Fry eggs in the oil and serve with the chips and brown sauce or tomato ketchup. Follow with the banana.

Snack   *75g/3oz grill chips or oven*   *15ml/1 tablespoon tomato*
chips   *ketchup*
2 slices bread, 40g/1½oz each
Cook chips as instructed on the packet. Make into a chip 'butty' or sandwich with the bread and tomato ketchup.

A CHOCOLATE-LOVER'S DAY

Milk allowance   *275ml/½ pint skimmed milk*
to use in tea or coffee

Breakfast   *25g/1 oz any bran breakfast*   *90ml/6 tablespoons skimmed*
cereal   *milk*
1 small banana

Light meal   *50g/2oz roast chicken or*   *45ml/3 tablespoons natural*
turkey   *yogurt*
2 sticks celery   *Few drops lemon juice*
1 medium apple   *Salt and pepper*
3 walnut halves
Discard any skin from chicken or turkey and cut flesh into small pieces. Chop celery. Core and dice apple. Roughly chop walnuts. Mix all ingredients together and season with salt and pepper.

Main meal *1 bacon or ham steak,*   *115g/4oz broccoli, frozen or*
    100g/3½oz   *fresh*
    1 pineapple ring, canned in   *1 choc-ice*
       natural juice, drained
    115g/4oz sweetcorn, frozen
       or canned
Grill bacon or ham steak. Heat pineapple under the grill.
Boil vegetables and serve with the steak and pineapple.
Follow with the choc-ice.

Snack 1 *50g/2oz bar chocolate*

Snack 2 *1 chocolate flake*

Snack 3 *150ml/¼ pint skimmed milk,*   *20ml/2 rounded teaspoons*
    extra to allowance   *drinking chocolate*

A SAVOURY SNACK-LOVER'S DAY

Milk allowance *275ml/½ pint skimmed milk*
    to use in tea or coffee

Breakfast *1 egg, size 3*   *5ml/1 level teaspoon low-fat*
    1 slice bread, 40g/1½oz   *spread*
Poach egg. Toast bread and top with low-fat spread and
egg.

Light meal *113g/4oz carton cottage*   *1 small packet crisps,*
    cheese, any flavour except   *25g/1oz, any flavour*
    'with Cheddar'   *1 medium banana*
    2 sticks celery
Eat cottage cheese with the celery and crisps. Follow with
the banana.

Main meal *4 fish fingers*   *15ml/1 tablespoon tomato*
    115g/4oz peas, frozen   *ketchup*
    115g/4oz runner beans, fresh *Individual carton fruit*
       or frozen   *yogurt, any flavour*
Grill fish fingers without added fat. Boil the vegetables and
serve with the fish and ketchup. Follow with the yogurt.

Snack 1   *1 small packet crisps, 25g/1oz, any flavour*

Snack 2   *1 small packet wholewheat crunchies*

Snack 3   *1 small packet corn snacks*

A BISCUIT-LOVER'S DAY

Milk allowance   *275ml/½ pint skimmed milk to use in tea or coffee throughout the day*

Breakfast	*25g/1oz any bran breakfast cereal*	*75ml/5 tablespoons skimmed milk, extra to allowance*
	15ml/1 tablespoon raisins or sultanas	

Light meal   *3 crispbreads*   *Cucumber*
75ml/3 level tablespoons   *1 medium pear or peach*
   curd cheese
Spread crispbreads with curd cheese and top with cucumber. Follow with fruit.

Main meal   *175g/6oz chicken breast*   *50ml/2floz gravy made with*
115g/4oz mushrooms   *instant gravy mix or*
115g/4oz peas, frozen   *powder and water*
Grill chicken breast and then discard skin. Poach mushrooms in a little water and boil peas.

Snack   *175g/6oz chocolate*   or   *190g/6½oz Marie, Osborne*
digestives, plain   *or rich tea biscuits*
digestives, Lincoln or
shortcake biscuits
Weigh out biscuits in the morning and eat them when you like throughout the day.

A CAKE-LOVER'S DAY

Milk allowance   *275ml/½ pint skimmed milk for use in drinks*

Breakfast 1 slice wholemeal bread, 40g/1½oz, toasted
10ml/2 level teaspoons low-fat spread

10ml/2 level teaspoons marmalade or jam

Light meal 1 wholemeal roll, 45g/1¾oz
15ml/1 level tablespoon curd cheese
25g/1oz ham sausage

15ml/1 level tablespoon sweet pickle or piccalilli
1 medium apple or pear

Split the roll and spread with the curd cheese. Fill with ham sausage and pickle. Follow with the fruit.

Main meal 150g/5oz cod or haddock fillet
5ml/1 level teaspoon low-fat spread
115g/4oz runner beans

115g/4oz carrots
15ml/1 tablespoon tomato ketchup
1 medium banana

Dot fish with low-fat spread and grill. Boil the vegetables and serve with the fish and ketchup. Follow with the banana.

Either
Home-made Cakes 40g/1½oz butter or margarine
40g/1½oz caster sugar
1 egg, size 3

40g/1½oz self-raising flour
25g/1oz raisins or sultanas or currants

Preheat oven to 190°C/375°F, gas mark 5. Cream butter or margarine and caster sugar until light and fluffy. Lightly beat the egg and then beat into the creamed mixture half at a time. Fold in the flour and the dried fruit. Divide between paper cake cases. Bake for 15-20 minutes. Cool on a wire rack (or eat warm).

Or 6 individual shop-bought jam tarts

Or 4 shop-bought cup cakes and 3 individual chocolate-coated swiss rolls

Calorie Swap-Shop

If you really don't like one of the foods suggested in the 30-Day Diet, check this list and see if you can swap it for another food which will keep your calorie consumption just the same.

Of course, when a particular food is part of a recipe it probably can't be swapped. But there is no reason why you shouldn't change the vegetables or fruit which are served with a meal or some of the cheeses and cold meats. Check quantities carefully, though. If you swap peas for sweetcorn you will only be allowed half the amount, but if you swap peas for runner beans you can double the quantity.

FRUIT

Swap this	for this	or	or
15ml/1 level tablespoon raisins or sultanas	2 prunes	2 dried apricots	75g/3oz raspberries or strawberries
30ml/2 level tablespoons raisins or sultanas	1 medium apple	5 dried apricots	75g/3oz grapes
1 medium apple	75g/3oz grapes	3 dessert plums	115g/4oz fresh cherries
1 small apple	1 medium peach or nectarine	1 kiwi fruit	50g/2oz black or white grapes
1 large orange	1 medium banana	2 medium peaches or nectarines	150g/5oz black grapes
½ grapefruit	1 mandarin or satsuma or tangerine	150g/5oz slice melon	75g/3oz raspberries or strawberries
1 medium orange	1 medium apple	2 kiwi fruits	225g/8oz fresh apricots
1 small orange	1 medium peach or nectarine	50g/2oz black or white grapes	150g/5oz raspberries or strawberries

115g/4oz grapes	1 small banana	2 kiwi fruits	1 large pear
6 grapes	1 mandarine or tangerine or satsuma	½ grapefruit	15ml/1 level tablespoon raisins or sultanas
1 small banana	115g/4oz grapes	4 Victoria dessert plums	25g/1oz dried dates
1 medium banana	2 medium pears	1 large orange	4 rings pineapple, canned in natural juice, drained
1 large banana	2 medium apples	50g/2oz dried prunes	225g/8oz fresh cherries
1 medium pear	1 medium peach or nectarine	150g/5oz blackberries or black currants	2 rings pineapple, canned in natural juice, drained
1 medium peach or nectarine	1 kiwi fruit	150g/5oz raspberries or strawberries	1 small orange
225g/8oz slice melon	115g/4oz strawberries or raspberries	115g/4oz fresh apricots	115g/4oz blackberries or blackcurrants
115g/4oz raspberries or strawberries	200g/7oz slice melon	115g/4oz fresh apricots	75g/3oz dessert gooseberries
50g/2oz raspberries or strawberries	½ grapefruit	1 Victoria dessert plum	115g/4oz slice melon
2 dried apricots	2 prunes	1 mandarin or satsuma or tangerine	½ grapefruit
3 prunes	3 dried apricots	15ml/1 level tablespoon raisins or sultanas	1 dried fig
6 prunes	6 dried apricots	25g/1oz dried dates with stones	115g/4oz black grapes
2 rings pineapple, canned in natural juice, drained	1 medium pear	1 medium peach or nectarine	1 small orange

VEGETABLES

Swap this	for this	or	or
115g/4oz peas, frozen	50g/2oz sweetcorn, fresh or frozen	115g/4oz frozen mixed vegetables	115g/4oz broad beans
50g/2oz peas, frozen	115g/4oz runner beans	115g/4oz broccoli	115g/4oz Brussels sprouts
115g/4oz oven chips or grill chips	200g/7oz potato, boiled or baked in its jacket	50g/2oz brown rice, weighed raw	50g/2oz wholewheat pasta, weighed raw
150g/5oz roast potato, cut in large chunks	225g/8oz potato, boiled or baked in its jacket	175g/6oz potato, boiled and mashed with 5ml/1 level teaspoon butter and 15ml/1 tablespoon skimmed milk	50g/2oz rice, white or brown, weighed raw
115g/4oz potato	25g/1oz pasta, white or wholewheat, weighed raw	25g/1oz rice, white or brown, weighed raw	115g/4oz sweetcorn
150g/5oz potato	150g/5oz sweetcorn	150g/5.3oz can baked beans in tomato sauce	115g/4oz peas and 115g/4oz broad beans
175g/6oz potato	40g/1½oz rice, brown or white, weighed raw	215g/7.6oz can spaghetti in tomato sauce	115g/4oz sweetcorn and 115g/4oz broad beans
115g/4oz carrots	115g/4oz swede	115g/4oz cabbage	75g/3oz broccoli
75g/3oz carrots	75g/3oz runner beans	75g/3oz cabbage	115g/4oz cauliflower
115g/4oz mushrooms	2 tomatoes	115g/4oz cauliflower	115g/4oz courgettes

1 grilled tomato	50g/2oz mushrooms	50g/2oz courgettes	50g/2oz bean sprouts
2 grilled tomatoes	115g/4oz mushrooms	115g/4oz courgettes	115g/4oz cauliflower
115g/4oz broccoli	115g/4oz runner beans	115g/4oz Brussels sprouts	115g/4oz spinach, weighed raw
115g/4oz runner beans	115g/4oz Brussels sprouts	115g/4oz broccoli	50g/2oz peas
75g/3oz runner beans	50g/2oz French beans, frozen	115g/4oz bean sprouts	2 medium courgettes
50g/2oz runner beans	115g/4oz courgettes	115g/4oz mushrooms	115g/4oz cauliflower
115g/4oz broad beans	115g/4oz peas	50g/2oz sweetcorn	115g/4oz frozen mixed vegetables
75g/3oz mixed vegetables, frozen	75g/3oz peas	115g/4oz French beans, frozen	75g/3oz broad beans
115g/4oz Brussels sprouts	75g/3oz leeks	115g/4oz runner beans	50g/2oz parsnips
75g/3oz Brussels sprouts	115g/4oz asparagus	150g/5oz courgettes	150g/5oz cauliflower
75g/3oz broccoli	115g/4oz asparagus	150g/5oz aubergine	115g/4oz Jerusalem artichokes, boiled
50g/2oz broccoli	115g/4oz mushrooms	115g/4oz courgettes	115g/4oz cauliflower
50g/2oz French beans, frozen	75g/3oz runner beans	115g/4oz asparagus	75g/3oz carrots
115g/4oz cauliflower	75g/3oz cabbage	75g/3oz carrots	115g/4oz courgettes
115g/4oz cabbage	115g/4oz carrots	115g/4oz swede	150g/5oz bean sprouts

2 medium courgettes	50g/2oz French beans, frozen	115g/4oz Jerusalem artichokes	75g/3oz runner beans
115g/4oz swede	115g/4oz carrots	115g/4oz turnip	115g/4oz cabbage
75g/3oz swede	115g/4oz cauliflower	50g/2oz French beans, frozen	75g/3oz cabbage
115g/4oz sweetcorn	115g/4oz potato	115g/4oz rice, brown or white weighed raw	150g/5oz peas and 115g/4oz carrots
75g/3oz sweetcorn	150g/5oz peas	75g/3oz potato	150g/5oz mixed vegetables, frozen
50g/2oz sweetcorn	115g/4oz broad beans	75g/3oz mixed vegetables	75g/3oz peas
115g/4oz bean sprouts	50g/2oz French beans, frozen	75g/3oz runner beans	75g/3oz broccoli
225g/7.9oz can baked beans in tomato sauce	215g/7.6oz can spaghetti in tomato sauce	175g/6oz potato	100g/3½oz oven or grill chips
215g/7.6oz can spaghetti in tomato sauce	225g/7.9oz can baked beans in tomato sauce	175g/6oz potato	100g/3½oz oven or grill chips
150g/5.3oz can baked beans in tomato sauce	115g/4oz sweetcorn	25g/1oz rice, brown or white, weighed raw	100g/4oz potato

FISH

Swap this	for this	or	or
3 fish fingers	2 salmon fish cakes	175g/6oz plaice fillet	175g/6oz trout

4 fish fingers	3 fish cakes		
175g/6oz trout	175g/6oz plaice fillet	200g/7oz cod or haddock fillet	130g/4½oz fresh salmon cutlet
50g/2oz prawns	40g/1½oz canned salmon	1 sardine, drained	50g/2oz tuna in brine, drained
115g/4oz prawns	75g/3oz crab meat	75g/3oz pilchards, canned in tomato sauce	100g/3½oz can tuna in brine
175g/6oz cod fillet	150g/5oz plaice fillet	175g/6oz haddock fillet	175g/6oz coley fillet
75g/3oz kipper fillet	1 whole herring, 130g/4½oz	175g/6oz smoked haddock fillet	3 fish cakes

MEAT

Swap this	for this	or	or
1 rasher bacon, well grilled	1 beef chipolata sausage, well grilled	25g/1oz lean cooked ham	25g/1oz ham sausage
2 rashers streaky bacon, well grilled	1 bacon or ham steak, 100g/3½oz raw, grilled	50g/2oz lean cooked ham	2 lamb's kidneys
50g/2oz lean cooked ham	40g/1½oz corned beef	50g/2oz ham sausage	70g/2½oz cooked turkey, no skin
50g/2oz corned beef	25g/1oz salami (Belgian, German or Hungarian)	75g/3oz roast chicken or turkey, no skin	70g/2½oz lean cooked ham
40g/1½oz corned beef	50g/2oz lean cooked ham	50g/2oz lean roast topside of beef	50g/2oz ham sausage
50g/2oz garlic sausage	25g/1oz salami, (Belgian, German or Hungarian)	25g/1oz Cervelat	75g/3oz lean roast topside of beef

50g/2oz lean roast top-side of beef	50g/2oz roast chicken, no skin	50g/2oz lean cooked ham	25g/1oz sausage
100g/3½oz lean roast topside of beef	115g/4oz roast turkey, no skin	75g/3oz lean roast leg of pork	75g/3oz lean roast leg of lamb
75g/3oz roast chicken, no skin	75g/3oz lean roast topside of beef	70g/2½oz lean roast leg of pork	70g/2½oz lean roast lamb
115g/4oz lean roast leg of lamb	115g/4oz lean roast leg of pork	1 chicken breast, 175g/6oz raw, grilled	1 gammon rasher, 150g/5oz raw, well grilled
75g/3oz gammon rasher, well grilled	1 large pork sausage, well grilled	2 chicken drumsticks, grilled and skin removed	75g/3oz rump steak, well grilled
Chicken leg joint, 225g/8oz raw, grilled and skin removed	2 rashers back bacon, well grilled	3 beef chipolata sausages, well grilled	75g/3oz lamb's liver, brushed with 5ml/1 teaspoon low-fat spread and grilled
175g/6oz pork chop well grilled	155g/5½oz lamb chump chop, well grilled	150g/5oz gammon rasher, well grilled	2 pork chipolatas well grilled and 2 rashers streaky bacon, well grilled
150g/5oz lamb loin chop, well grilled	3 pork and beef chipolata sausages, well grilled	200g/7oz chicken breast, grilled and skin removed	50g/2oz lamb's liver grilled and 1 rasher back bacon, well grilled
115g/4oz minute steak, grilled	250g/9oz chicken leg joint, grilled and skin removed	2 beefburgers, 50g/2oz each, well grilled	4 rashers streaky bacon, well grilled

115g/4oz lamb's liver, grilled	2 lamb's kidneys, grilled and 2 beef chipolata sausages well grilled	2 bacon or ham steaks, 100g/3½oz each, well grilled	150g/5oz pork fillet, lean only, cut into cubes and threaded on a skewer, and grilled
1 beef chipolata sausage, well grilled	1 rasher streaky bacon, well grilled	1 lamb's kidney, grilled	25g/1oz lean cooked ham
2 beef chipolata sausages, well grilled	2 rashers streaky bacon well grilled	1 bacon steak, 100g/3½oz raw, well grilled	2 lamb's kidneys, grilled
50g/2oz liver pâté	50g/2oz garlic sausage	50g/2oz liver sausage	75g/3oz smoked ham sausage

CHEESE

Swap this	*for this*	*or*	*or*
1 triangle cheese spread	30ml/2 level tablespoons curd cheese	45ml/3 level tablespoons cottage cheese	15ml/1 level tablespoon cheese spread
2 triangles cheese spread	50g/2oz curd cheese	75g/3oz cottage cheese, with chives, onion or pineapple	25g/1oz Edam or Tendale
25g/1oz Edam or Tendale	25g/1oz Camembert or Brie	25g/1oz Austrian Smoked or Bavarian Smoked	50g/2oz curd cheese
40g/1½oz Edam or Tendale	25g/1oz Cheddar or Gruyère	35g/1¼oz Cotswold or Double Gloucester or Leicester	113g/4oz carton cottage cheese with Cheddar & Onion

50g/2oz Edam or Tendale	40g/1½oz Cheddar	45g/1¾oz Dolcellata or Samsoe or Gouda	50g/2oz Camembert or Brie
45g/1¾oz Camembert	40g/1½oz Cotswold or Double Gloucester or Leicester	113g/4oz carton curd cheese	75g/3oz Feta or Riccotta
113g/4oz carton curd cheese	40g/1½oz Danish Blue or Leicester or Lymeswold	150g/5oz cottage cheese with salmon & cucumber	40g/1½oz Cheshire or Lancashire
50g/2oz cottage cheese	15ml/1 level tablespoon cheese spread	30ml/2 level tablespoons curd cheese	15g/½oz Leicester, Cotswold or Double Gloucester

Calorie Chart of Basic Foods

Exact metric conversions have been given in the chart below. In the recipes in the main part of the book, and with portions below, the metric equivalents have been rounded off for convenience.

ALMONDS

Shelled, per 28g/1oz	160
Ground, per 15ml/1 level tablespoon	30
Per almond, whole	10
Per sugared almond	15

ANCHOVIES

Per 28g/1oz	40
Per anchovy fillet	5

ANCHOVY PASTE OR ESSENCE

Per 5ml/1 level teaspoon	5

ANGELICA

Per 28g/1oz	90
Per stick	10

APPLES

Cooking, per 28g/1oz	10
Eating, per 28g/1oz	13
Medium whole eating, 150g/5oz	65
Medium whole cooking, 225g/8oz	80
Apple sauce, sweetened, per 15ml/1 level tablespoon	20
Apple sauce, unsweetened, per 15ml/1 level tablespoon	10

APRICOTS
Per 28g/1oz unless otherwise stated

Canned in natural juice	13
Canned in syrup	30
Dried	52
Fresh with stone	7
Per dried apricot	10
Per apricot half, canned in syrup	15
Per whole fresh fruit	5

ARROWROOT

Per 28g/1oz	101
Per 5ml/1 level teaspoon	10

ARTICHOKES

Globe, boiled, per 28g/1oz	4
1 medium globe artichoke	10
Jerusalem, boiled, 28g/1oz	5

ASPARAGUS

Raw or boiled, per 28g/1oz	5
Per asparagus spear	5

AUBERGINES

Raw, per 28g/1oz	4
Sliced, fried, 28g/1oz raw weight	60
Whole aubergine, 200g/7oz	28
Whole aubergine, sliced, fried, 200g/7oz raw weight	405

AVOCADO

Flesh only, per 28g/1oz	63
Per half avocado, 105g/3¾oz	235

BACON
Per 28g/1oz unless otherwise stated

Back rasher, raw	122
Collar joint, raw, lean and fat	91
Collar joint, boiled, lean only	54
Collar joint, boiled, lean and fat	92
Streaky rashers, raw	118
1 streaky rasher, well grilled or fried, 20g/¾oz raw weight	50
1 back rasher, well grilled or fried, 35g/1¼oz raw weight	80
1 bacon steak, well grilled, 100g/3½oz raw weight	105

BAKING POWDER

Per 28g/1oz	46
Per 5ml/1 level teaspoon	5

BANANAS

Flesh only, per 28g/1oz	22
Flesh and skin, per 28g/1oz	13
Small whole fruit, 150g/5oz	65
Medium whole fruit, 175g/6oz	80
Large whole fruit, 200g/7oz	95
Whole fruit, peeled, fried in batter, 175g/6oz raw weight	170
Dried, per 28g/1oz	140

BARCELONA NUTS

Shelled, per 28g/1oz	181

BARLEY, PEARL

Raw, per 28g/1oz	102
Boiled, per 28g/1oz	34
Per 15ml/1 level tablespoon, raw	45

BARLEY CUP

Per 28g/1oz	80

BASS

Fillet, steamed, per 28g/1oz	35

BEAN SPROUTS

Canned, per 28g/1oz	3
Raw, per 28g/1oz	5
Boiled, per 28g/1oz	7

BEANS
Per 28g/1oz

Aduki, raw weight	92
Baked, canned in tomato sauce	20
Black eye, raw weight	93
Broad, boiled	14
Butter, boiled	27
Butter, raw weight	77
Cannellini, canned	25
French, frozen	10
Haricot, boiled	26
Haricot, raw weight	77
Lima, raw, dry weight	92
Mung, raw, dry weight	92
Red kidney, canned	25
Red kidney, raw, dry weight	77
Runner, boiled	5
Runner, raw	7
Snap, raw, green	10
Soya, raw, dry weight	115

BEECH NUTS

Shelled, per 28g/1oz	160

BEEF
Per 28g/1oz unless otherwise stated

Brisket, boiled, lean and fat	92
Brisket, raw, lean and fat	71
Fillet steak, medium grilled, 175g/6oz	305
Ground beef, lean, raw	45
Ground beef, lean, fried and drained of fat	55
Ground beef, lean, fried and drained of fat, 28g/1oz raw weight	40
Minced beef, raw	74
Minced beef, well fried and drained of fat	82
Minced beef, well fried and drained of fat, 28g/1oz raw weight	59
Rump steak, fried, lean only	54
Rump steak, grilled, lean only	48
Rump steak, raw, lean and fat	56
Rump steak, well grilled, 175g/6oz raw	260
Rump steak, medium grilled, 175g/6oz raw	290
Rump steak, rare grilled, 175g/6oz raw	310
Silverside, salted, boiled, lean and fat	69
Silverside, salted, boiled, lean only	49
Sirloin, roast, lean and fat	80
Sirloin, roast, lean only	55
Stewing steak, raw, lean only	35
Stewing steak, raw, lean and fat	50
Stewing steak, stewed, lean and fat	63
Topside, raw, lean only	35
Topside, raw, lean and fat	51
Topside, roast, lean and fat	61
Topside, roast, lean only	44

BEETROOT

Raw, per 28g/1oz	8
Boiled, per 28g/1oz	12
Per baby beet, boiled	5

BILBERRIES

Raw or frozen, per 28g/1oz	16

BLACKBERRIES

Raw or frozen, per 28g/1oz	8
Stewed, without sugar, per 28g/1oz	7

BLACKCURRANTS

Raw or frozen, per 28g/1oz	8
Stewed, without sugar, per 28g/1oz	7
Canned in syrup, per 28g/1oz	23

BLACK PUDDING

Raw, per 28g/1oz	78
Sliced and fried, 28g/1oz raw weight	85

BLOATERS

Fillet, grilled, per 28g/1oz	71
On the bone, grilled, per 28g/1oz	53

BRAINS
Per 28g/1oz

Calves' and lambs', raw	31
Calves' boiled	43
Lambs' boiled	36

BRAN
Per 28g/1oz

	58
Per 15ml/1 level tablespoon	10

BRANDY BUTTER

Per 28g/1oz	170

BRAWN

Per 28g/1oz	43

BRAZIL NUTS

Shelled, per 28g/1oz	175
Per nut	20
Per buttered Brazil	40
Per chocolate Brazil	55

BREAD
Per 28g/1oz

Black Rye	90
Bran	65
Brown or Wheatmeal	63
Currant	71
Enriched, eg Cholla	110
Fried bread, 28g/1oz unfried weight	160
French	65
Fruit Sesame	120
Granary	70
Light Rye	70
Malt	70
Milk	80
Pumpernickel	60
Soda	75
Vogel	65
Wheatgerm, eg Hovis and Vitbe	65
White	66
Wholemeal (100%)	61

Per slice white bread from a sliced loaf

Thin slice from a large loaf	75
Thin slice from a long loaf	60
Medium slice from a small loaf	60
Medium slice from a large loaf	85
Medium slice from a long loaf	75
Thick slice from a large loaf	100
Thick slice from a long loaf	90

Per slice brown or wheatmeal bread from a sliced loaf

Medium slice from a small loaf	55
Medium slice from a large loaf	80
Medium slice from a long loaf	75

Per slice wholemeal bread from a sliced loaf

Medium slice from a small loaf	55
Medium slice from a large loaf	75
Medium slice from a long loaf	70

Rolls, buns, etc. each

Baby bridge roll, 15g/½oz	35
Bagel, 40g/1½oz	150
Bap, 40g/1½oz	130
Bath bun, 40g/1½oz	120
Bread stick	15
Brioche roll, 45g/1¾oz	215
Chelsea bun, 90g/3¼oz	255
Croissant, 40g/1½oz	165
Croissant, 65g/2½oz	280
Crumpet, 40g/1½oz	75
Crusty roll, brown or white, 45g/1¾oz	145
Currant bun, 45g/1¾oz	150
Devonshire split, 65g/2½oz	195
Dinner roll, 40g/1½oz	130
French toast, average slice	50
Hot cross bun, 50g/2oz	180
Hovis roll, 45g/1¾oz	115
Morning roll, Aberdeen	185
Muffin, 60g/2¼oz	125
Pitta, 65g/2½oz	205
Scone, plain, 50g/2oz	210
Soft brown roll, 45g/1¾oz	140
Soft white roll, 45g/1¾oz	155
Tea cake, 50g/2oz	155
Wholemeal roll, 45g/1¾oz	125

Per 15ml/1 level tablespoon

Breadcrumbs, dried	30
Breadcrumbs, fresh	8
Bread sauce	15

BROCCOLI

Raw, per 28g/1oz	7
Boiled, per 28g/1oz	5

BRUSSELS SPROUTS

Raw, per 28g/1oz	7
Boiled, per 28g/1oz	5

BUCKWHEAT

Whole grain, per 28g/1oz	99

BUTTER

All brands, per 28g/1oz	210
Per 15ml/1 level tablespoon	105

CABBAGE

Raw, per 28g/1oz	6
Boiled, per 28g/1oz	4

Per 15ml/1 level tablespoon

Pickled red	3
Sauerkraut	5

CANDY FLOSS

Per 28g/1oz	80
Per medium stick	60

CAPERS

Per 28g/1oz	5

CARROTS

Raw, per 28g/1oz	6
Boiled, per 28g/1oz	5
Per average carrot, 50g/2oz	12
Sliced, fried, 28g/1oz raw weight	30

CASHEW NUTS

Shelled, per 28g/1oz	167
Per nut	15

CASSAVA

Fresh, per 28g/1oz	43

CAULIFLOWER

Raw, per 28g/1oz	4
Boiled, per 28g/1oz	3

CAVIAR

Per 28g/1oz	75

CELERIAC

Raw, per 28g/1oz	8
Boiled, per 28g/1oz	4

CELERY

Raw, per 28g/1oz	2
Boiled, per 28g/1oz	1
Per stick of celery	5

CHEESE
Per 28g/1oz

Appenzell	113
Austrian Smoked	78
Babybel	97
Bavarian Smoked	80
Bel Paese	96
Blue Stilton	131
Bonbel	102
Boursin	116
Bresse Bleu	80
Brie	88
Caerphilly	120
Caithness Morven	110
Caithness Full Fat Soft	110
Camembert	88
Cheddar	120
Cheese spread	80
Cheshire	110
Cheviot	120
Cotswold	105
Cottage cheese	27
Cream cheese	124
Curd cheese	54
Danbo	98
Danish Blue	103
Danish Elbo	98
Danish Esrom	98
Danish Fynbo	100
Danish Havarti	117
Danish Maribo	100
Danish Molbo	100
Danish Mozzarella	98
Danish Mycella	99

Danish Saga	98
Danish Samsoe	98
Derby	110
Dolcellata	100
Double Gloucester	105
Edam	88
Emmenthal	115
Fetta	54
Gorgonzola	112
Gouda	100
Gruyère	117
Halumi	84
Ilchester	112
Jarlsberg	95
Lancashire	109
Leicester	105
Lymeswold	120
Norwegian Blue	100
Norwegian Gjeost	133
Orangerulle	92
Orkney Claymore	111
Parmesan	118
Philadelphia	90
Port Salut	94
Processed	88
Rambol, with walnuts	117
Red Windsor	119
Riccotta	55
Roquefort	88
Royalp	110
Sage Derby	112
Skimmed milk soft cheese	25
Sprinz	124
St Paulin	98
Tendale	70
Tome au Raisin	74
Wensleydale	115
White Stilton	96

Per 15ml/1 level tablespoon

Cheese spread	50
Cottage cheese	15
Cream cheese	60
Curd cheese	20
Parmesan cheese, grated	30

CHERRIES

Fresh, with stones, per 28g/1oz	12
Glacé, per 28g/1oz	60
Per glacé cherry	10
Per cocktail cherry	10

CHESTNUTS

Shelled, per 28g/1oz	48
With shells	40
Chestnut purée, sweetened, per 28g/1oz	25

CHICK PEAS

Raw, per 28g/1oz	91

CHICKEN
Per 28g/1oz unless otherwise stated

On the bone, raw	25
Meat only, raw	34
Meat only, boiled	52

Meat only, roast	42
Meat and skin, roast	61
Chicken breast, fried, 175g/6oz average raw weight	215
Chicken breast, fried and skin removed, 175g/6oz average raw weight	150
Chicken breast, grilled, 175g/6oz average raw weight	200
Chicken breast, grilled and skin removed, 175g/6oz average raw weight	145
Chicken drumstick, raw, 100g/3½oz	90
Chicken drumstick, fried, 100g/3½oz average raw weight	105
Chicken drumstick, fried in egg and breadcrumbs, 100g/3½oz average raw weight	130
Chicken drumstick, grilled and skin removed, 100g/3½oz average raw weight	65
Chicken drumstick, grilled 100g/3½oz average raw weight	85
Chicken leg joint, raw, 225g/8oz average weight	410
Chicken leg joint, raw, skin removed, 225g/8oz average weight	165
Chicken leg joint, grilled, 225g/8oz raw weight	250
Chicken leg joint, grilled and skin removed, 225g/8oz raw weight	165
Chicken leg joint, roasted, 225g/8oz raw weight	290
Chicken leg joint, roasted and skin removed, 225g/8oz raw weight	190
Chicken leg joint, fried, 225g/8oz raw weight	285
Chicken leg joint, fried and skin removed, 225g/8oz raw weight	175
Chicken leg joint, fried in egg and breadcrumbs, 225g/8oz raw weight	435
Chicken leg joint, poached in stock, skin removed, 225g/8oz raw weight	165

CHICORY

Raw, per 28g/1oz	3
Essence, per 28g/1oz	60

CHILLIES

Dried, per 28g/1oz	85

CHIVES

Per 28g/1oz	10

CHINESE LEAVES

Raw, per 28g/1oz	3
Boiled, per 28g/1oz	2

CHOCOLATE
Per 28g/1oz

Milk or Plain	150
Cooking	155
Vermicelli	135

Per 5ml/1 level teaspoon

Vermicelli	20

CLAMS

With shells, raw, per 28g/1oz	15
Without shells, raw, per 28g/1oz	25

COB NUTS

With shells, per 28g/1oz	39
Shelled, per 28g/1oz	108
Per nut	5

COCKLES

Without shells, boiled, per 28g/1oz	14

COCOA POWDER

Per 28g/1oz	89
Per 5ml/1 level teaspoon	10

COCONUT
Per 28g/1oz unless otherwise stated

Fresh	100
Desiccated	171
Desiccated, per 15ml/1 level tablespoon	30
Coconut milk, per 28ml/1floz	6
Creamed coconut	218

COD
Per 28g/1oz unless otherwise stated

Fillet, raw	22
Fillet, baked or grilled with a little fat	27
Fillet, in batter, fried	56
Fillet, poached in water or steamed	24
Frozen steaks, raw	19
On the bone, raw	15
Fillet in batter, deep fried, 175g/6oz raw unbattered weight	460

COD LIVER OIL

Per 5ml/1 teaspoon	40

COD ROE

Hard roe, raw	32
Hard roe, fried in egg and breadcrumbs	55

COFFEE
Per 28g/1oz

Fresh, infused	0
Instant	28
Coffee and chicory essence	62
Instant coffee, per 10ml/1 rounded teaspoon	0

COLEY
Per 28g/1oz

Fillet, raw	21
On bone, steamed	24
Fillet, steamed	28

CORNED BEEF

Per 28g/1oz	62

CORNFLOUR

Per 28g/1oz	100
Per 15ml/1 level tablespoon	33

CORN OIL

Per 28g/1oz	255
Per 15ml/1 tablespoon	120

CORN ON THE COB

Average whole cob	155

COUGH SYRUP

Thick, per 5ml/1 teaspoon	15
Thin, per 5ml/1 teaspoon	5

COURGETTES

Raw, per 28g/1oz	4
Per courgette, 65g/2½oz	10
Sliced, fried, 28g/1oz raw weight	15

CRAB

With shell, per 28g/1oz boiled	7

Meat only, per 28g/1oz boiled — 36
Average crab with shell — 95

CRANBERRIES
Raw, per 28g/1oz — 4

CRANBERRY SAUCE
Per 28g/1oz — 65
Per 15ml/1 level tablespoon — 45

CREAM
Per 28g/1oz
Clotted — 165
Double — 127
Half cream — 35
Imitation — 85
Single — 60
Soured — 60
Sterilized, canned — 65
Whipping — 94
Per 15ml/1 level tablespoon
Clotted — 105
Double — 56
Half — 20
Imitation — 55
Single — 30
Soured — 30
Sterilized, canned — 35
Whipping — 45

CUCUMBER
Raw, per 28g/1oz — 3

CURRANTS
Per 28g/1oz — 69
Per 15ml/1 level tablespoon — 20

CURRY PASTE
Per 28g/1oz — 40

CURRY POWDER
Per 28g/1oz — 66
Per 5ml/1 level teaspoon — 12

CUSTARD APPLE
Flesh only, raw, per 28g/1oz — 25

CUSTARD POWDER
Per 28g/1oz — 100
Per 15ml/1 level tablespoon — 33

CUSTARD
Per 150ml/¼ pint, made as instructed with Silver Top milk — 175
Per 150ml/¼pt, made as instructed with skimmed milk — 130

DAMSONS
Fresh, with stones, per 28g/1oz — 11
Stewed, no sugar, per 28g/1oz — 8

DATES
Per 28g/1oz
Dried, with stones — 60
Dried, without stones — 70
Fresh with stones — 30
Chopped and sugar rolled — 77
Per date, fresh — 15

DELICATESSEN SAUSAGES
Per 28g/1oz
Belgian Liver Sausage — 90
Bierwurst — 75
Bockwurst — 180
Cervelat — 140
Chorizo — 140
Continental Liver Sausage — 85

Frankfurter — 78
French Garlic Sausage — 90
Garlic Sausage — 70
Ham Sausage — 50
Kabanos — 115
Krakowska — 80
Liver Sausage — 88
Mettwurst — 120
Mortadella, Italian — 105
Pastrami — 65
Polish Country Sausage — 60
Polony — 80
Pork Boiling Ring, coarse — 110
Salami, Belgian — 130
Salami, Danish — 160
Salami, Hungarian — 130
Salami, German — 120
Saveloy — 74
Smoked Dutch Sausage — 105
Smoked Pork Sausage — 130
Smoked Ham Sausage — 65

DOGFISH
Fried in batter, per 28g/1oz — 75

DRIPPING
Per 28g/1oz — 253
Per 15ml/1 level tablespoon — 125

DUCK
Per 28g/1oz
Raw, meat only — 35
Raw, meat, fat and skin — 122
Roast, meat only — 54
Roast, meat, fat and skin — 96

DUCK EGGS
Per average egg, 99g/3½oz — 170

EEL
Meat only, raw, per 28g/1oz — 48
Meat only, stewed, per 28g/1oz — 57
Jellied eels plus some jelly, 85g/3oz — 180
Smoked, per 28g/1oz — 55

EGGS each	raw	fried
Size 1	95	115
Size 2	90	110
Size 3	80	100
Size 4	75	95
Size 5	70	90
Size 6	60	80
Yolk of size 3 egg	65	
White of size 3 egg	15	

ENDIVE
Raw, per 28g/1oz — 3

FENNEL
Raw, per 28g/1oz — 6
Boiled, per 28g/1oz — 8

FIGS
Dried, per 28g/1oz — 60
Fresh, green, per 28g/1oz — 12
Per dried fig — 30

FLOUR
Per 28g/1oz
Wheatmeal — 93
White, plain — 99

White, self-raising — 96
White, strong — 96
Wholemeal — 90
Buckwheat — 99
Cassava — 97
Granary — 99
Maizemeal or Cornmeal (96%) — 103
Maizemeal or Cornmeal (60%) — 100
Rice — 100
Rye (100%) — 95
Soya, low-fat — 100
Soya, full fat — 127
Yam — 90
Per 15ml/1 level tablespoon
White — 32
Wholemeal — 29

FLOUNDER
On the bone; raw, per 28g/1oz — 20
On the bone, steamed, per 28g/1oz — 15

FRENCH DRESSING
Per 15ml/1 tablespoon — 75

FRUIT
Crystallised, per 28g/1oz — 75

GAMMON
Per 28g/1oz
Gammon joint, raw, lean and fat — 67
Gammon joint, boiled, lean and fat — 76
Gammon joint, boiled, lean — 47
Gammon rashers, grilled, lean and fat — 65
Gammon rashers, grilled, lean — 49
Gammon rasher, well grilled, 175g/6oz raw — 260

GARLIC
One clove — 0

GELATINE
Per 28g/1oz — 96
Per 15ml/1 level tablespoon — 30
Per envelope, 10g — 35

GHEE
Per 28g/1oz — 235

GHERKINS
Per 28g/1oz — 5

GINGER
Ground, per 28g/1oz — 73
Ground, per 5ml/1 level teaspoon — 8
Root, raw, peeled, per 28g/1oz — 18
Stem, in syrup, drained, per 28g/1oz — 60
Stem in syrup, drained, per medium piece — 40
Syrup from stem ginger, per 28g/1oz — 55

GOOSE
Roast, on the bone, per 28g/1oz — 55
Roast, meat only (without skin), per 28g/1oz — 90

GOOSEBERRIES
Fresh, ripe dessert, per 28g/1oz — 10
Fresh, cooking, per 28g/1oz — 5
Canned in syrup, per 28g/1oz — 22

GRAPEFRUIT
Per 28g/1oz unless otherwise stated
Canned in natural juice — 11

Item	Value
Canned in syrup	17
Flesh only	6
Flesh and skin	3
Medium whole fruit, 350g/12oz	35
Juice, unsweetened, per 28ml/1floz	9
Juice, unsweetened, per 150ml/¼ pint	45
Juice, sweetened, per 150ml/¼ pint	55
GRAPES	
Black, per 28g/1oz	14
White, per 28g/1oz	17
Per grape	4
GRAVY	
Per 30ml/2 tablespoons	
Thick, made with meat dripping	30
Thick, made without fat	10
Thin, made without fat	5
GREENGAGES	
Fresh, with stones, per 28g/1oz	13
Stewed, with stones, no sugar, per 28g/1oz	11
GRENADINE SYRUP	
Per 28g/1oz	72
GROUSE	
Roast, meat only, per 28g/1oz	50
GROUND RICE	
Per 28g/1oz	100
Per 15ml/1 level tablespoon	33
GUAVAS	
Fresh, with seeds, per 28g/1oz	16
Canned, per 28g/1oz	17
GUINEA FOWL	
Roast, on the bone, per 28g/1oz	30
Roast, meat only, per 28g/1oz	60
HADDOCK	
Per 28g/1oz unless otherwise stated	
Fillet, raw	21
Fillet in breadcrumbs, fried	50
On the bone, raw	15
On the bone, in breadcrumbs, fried	45
Smoked fillet, steamed or poached in water	29
Fillet in breadcrumbs, fried, 175g/6oz raw weight	435
Fillet in batter, deep fried, 175g/6oz raw weight	460
HAGGIS	
Cooked, per 28g/1oz	89
HAKE	
Per 28g/1oz	
Fillet, raw	20
Fillet, steamed	30
Fillet, fried	60
On the bone, raw	10
HALIBUT	
Per 28g/1oz	
Fillet, steamed	37
On the bone, raw	26
On the bone, steamed	28
HAM	
Per 28g/1oz unless otherwise stated	
Chopped ham roll or loaf	75
Ham, boiled, lean	47
Ham, boiled, fatty	90
Honey roast ham	50
Old Smokey ham	65
Maryland ham	55
Virginia ham	40
Ham steak, well grilled, 100g/3½oz average raw weight	105
HARE	
Stewed, meat only, per 28g/1oz	54
Stewed, on bone, per 28g/1oz	39
HASLET	
Per 28g/1oz	80
HAZEL NUTS	
Shelled, per 28g/1oz	108
Per nut	5
HEART	
Per 28g/1oz unless otherwise stated	
Lamb's, raw	34
Ox, raw	31
Pig's, raw	26
Whole lamb's heart, roasted, 115g/4oz average raw weight	270
HERRING	
Per 28g/1oz unless otherwise stated	
Fillet, raw	66
Fillet, grilled	56
Fillet in oatmeal, fried	66
On the bone, grilled	38
On the bone in oatmeal, fried	59
Rollmop herring	47
Average rollmop herring, 70g/2½oz weight	120
Whole herring, grilled, 130g/4½oz raw weight	170
HERRING ROE	
Fried, per 28g/1oz	69
Soft roe, raw, per 28g/1oz	23
HONEY	
Per 28g/1oz	82
Per 5ml/1 level teaspoon	20
HORSERADISH	
Fresh root, per 28g/1oz	17
Horseradish sauce, per 15ml/1 level tablespoon	13
HUMUS	
Per 28g/1oz	50
HUNDREDS AND THOUSANDS	
Per 5ml/1 level teaspoon	15
ICE CREAM	
Per 28g/1oz	
Soft ice cream (eg Mr Whippy)	45
Vanilla	47
ICING	
Royal, per 28g/1oz	85
JAM	
Per 28g/1oz	74
Per 5ml/1 level teaspoon	15
JELLY	
As sold, per 28g/1oz	73
Made up with water, 150ml/¼ pint	85
Per cube	29
KIDNEY	
All types, raw, per 28g/1oz	26
Lamb's kidney, grilled, 50g/2oz average raw weight	50
Lamb's kidney, fried, 50g/2oz average raw weight	65
KIPPERS	
Fillet, baked or grilled, per 28g/1oz	58
On the bone, baked, per 28g/1oz	32
Whole kipper, grilled, 175g/6oz raw weight	280
KIWI FRUIT	
1 medium	30
LAMB	
Per 28g/1oz unless otherwise stated	
Breast, boned, raw, lean and fat	107
Breast, boned, roast, lean and fat	116
Breast, boned, roast, lean only	71
Leg, raw, lean and fat, without bone	68
Leg, raw, lean only, without bone	46
Leg, roast, lean and fat, without bone	75
Leg, roast, lean, without bone	54
Scrag and neck, raw, lean and fat, weighed with bone	54
Scrag and neck, raw, lean and fat, weighed without bone	90
Scrag and neck, stewed, lean only, weighed with bone	38
Scrag and neck, stewed, lean only, weighed without bone	72
Scrag and neck, stewed, lean and fat, weighed without bone	83
Shoulder, boned, raw, lean and fat	89
Shoulder, boned, roast, lean	56
Chump chop, well grilled, 150g/5oz raw weight	205
Loin chop, well grilled, 150g/5oz raw weight	175
LARD	
Per 28g/1oz	253
Per 15ml/1 level tablespoon	125
LAVERBREAD	
Per 28g/1oz	15
LEEKS	
Raw, per 28g/1oz	9
Average whole leek, raw	25
LEMON	
Flesh and skin, per 28g/1oz	4
Lemon juice, per 15ml/1 tablespoon	0
LEMON CURD	
Per 28g/1oz	80
Per 5ml/1 level teaspoon	15
LEMON SOLE	
Per 28g/1oz	
Fillet, steamed or poached	26
On the bone, steamed or poached	18
LENTILS	
Raw, per 28g/1oz	86
Boiled, per 28g/1oz	28
LETTUCE	
Fresh, per 28g/1oz	3
LIVER	
Per 28g/1oz unless otherwise stated	
Chicken's, raw	38
Chicken's, fried	55

Food	Calories
Lamb's, raw	51
Lamb's, fried	66
Ox, raw	46
Ox, stewed	56
Pig's, raw	44
Pig's, stewed	54
Liver sausage	88
Lamb's, fried, 115g/4oz raw weight	235
Lamb's, grilled without fat, 115g/4oz raw weight	205

LOBSTER
With shell, boiled, per 28g/1oz	12
Meat only, boiled, per 28g/1oz	34

LOGANBERRIES
Fresh, per 28g/1oz	5
Canned in syrup, per 28g/1oz	29

LOW FAT SPREAD
All brands, eg Outline, St Ivel Gold, per 28g/1oz	105
Per 5ml/1 level teaspoon	15

LUNCHEON MEAT
Per 28g/1oz	89

LYCHEES
Fresh, flesh only, per 28g/1oz	18
Canned, per 28g/1oz	19
Per lychee	8

MACARONI
Raw, per 28g/1oz	105
Boiled, per 28g/1oz	33
Wholewheat macaroni, raw, per 28g/1oz	95
Wholewheat macaroni, boiled, per 28g/1oz	34

MACEDONIA NUTS
Shelled, per 28g/1oz	188

MACKEREL
Per 28g/1oz unless otherwise stated
Fillet, raw	63
Fillet, fried	53
On the bone, fried	39
Kippered mackerel	62
Smoked mackerel	70
Whole raw mackerel, 225g/8oz	320

MAIZE
Whole grain, per 28g/1oz	103

MANDARINS
Canned, per 28g/1oz	16
Fresh, with skin, per 28g/1oz	7
Whole fruit, 70g/2½oz	20

MANGO
Raw, per 28g/1oz	17
Canned, per 28g/1oz	22
Medium whole mango, 285g/10oz	100
Mango chutney, per 15ml/1 level tablespoon	35

MAPLE SYRUP
Per 28g/1oz	70

MARGARINE
All brands except those labelled "low fat", per 28g/1oz	210
Per 5ml/1 level teaspoon	35

MARMALADE
Per 28g/1oz	74
Per 5ml/1 level teaspoon	15

MARRON GLACE
Per 28g/1oz	74
One medium marron glacé	45

MARROW
Raw, per 28g/1oz	5
Boiled, per 28g/1oz	2

MARZIPAN (Almond Paste)
Per 28g/1oz	126
Petit Fours, per 28g/1oz	126

MAYONNAISE
Per 28g/1oz	205
Per 15ml/1 level tablespoon	95

MEDLARS
Flesh only, per 28g/1oz	12

MELON
Per 28g/1oz
Cantaloupe, with skin	4
Honeydew or Yellow, with skin	4
Ogen, with skin	5
Watermelon, with skin	3
Melon seeds, coat removed, per 28g/1oz	165
Slice of Cantaloupe, Honeydew or Yellow, with skin, 225g/8oz	30

MERINGUE
Shells, unfilled, per 28g/1oz	108

MILK
Per 568ml/1 pint
Buttermilk	232
Channel Island or Gold Top	445
Evaporated milk, full cream, reconstituted	360
Goat's	415
Homogenized or Red Top	380
Instant spray dried low-fat skimmed milk, reconstituted	200
Instant dried skimmed milk with vegetable fat, reconstituted	280
Longlife or UHT	380
Pasteurized or Silver Top	380
Pasteurized or Silver Top with cream removed, 500ml/18floz	240
Semi-skimmed milk	300
Skimmed or separated	195
Soya milk, diluted as directed	370
Sterilized	380
Untreated farm milk or Green Top	370

Per 15ml/1 tablespoon
Channel Island or Gold Top	12
Condensed, full cream, sweetened	50
Condensed, skimmed, sweetened	41
Evaporated full cream	23
Homogenized, Pasteurized, Green Top, Silver Top and Sterilized	10
Instant low-fat milk, dry	18
Instant low-fat milk, reconstituted	5
Skimmed or separated	5

Canned milk, per 28g/1oz
Evaporated full fat milk	45
Condensed, skimmed, sweetened	76
Condensed, full fat, sweetened	91
Condensed, unsweetened	40

MINCEMEAT
Per 28g/1oz	67
Per 15ml/1 level tablespoon	40

MINCE PIE
Medium pie, 50g/2oz	250

MINT
Fresh, per 28g/1oz	3

MINT SAUCE
Per 15ml/1 tablespoon	5

MIXED PEEL, CANDIED
Per 28g/1oz	90

MOLASSES
Per 28g/1oz	78
Per 15ml/1 tablespoon	45

MOULI
Raw, flesh only, per 28g/1oz	5

MUESLI
Per 28g/1oz	105
Per 15ml/1 level tablespoon	30

MULBERRIES
Raw, per 28g/1oz	10

MULLET
Raw, per 28g/1oz	40

MUSHROOMS
Raw, per 28g/1oz	4
Button, fried whole, 50g/2oz raw weight	80
Button, sliced and fried, 50g/2oz raw weight	100
Flat, fried whole, 50g/2oz raw weight	120
Flat, sliced and fried, 50g/2oz raw weight	150

MUSSELS
With shells, boiled, per 28g/1oz	7
Without shells, boiled, per 28g/1oz	25

MUSTARD & CRESS
Raw, per 28g/1oz	3
Whole carton	5

MUSTARD
Dry, per 28g/1oz	128
Made, English, per 5ml/1 level teaspoon	10
French, per 5ml/1 level teaspoon	10

NECTARINES
Fresh, with stone	13
Medium whole nectarine, 115g/4oz	50

NOODLES
Cooked, per 28g/1oz	33

NUTMEG
Powdered, per 2.5ml/½ level teaspoon	0

OATMEAL
Raw, per 28g/1oz	114
Per 15ml/1 level tablespoon, raw	40

OATS
Rolled, per 28g/1oz	115

OCTOPUS
Raw, per 28g/1oz	20

OKRA (Ladies' fingers)
Raw, per 28g/1oz	5

OLIVE OIL
Per 28g/1oz	255
Per 15ml/1 tablespoon	120

OLIVES
Stoned, in brine, per 28g/1oz	29

With stones, in brine, per 28g/1oz 23

Per stuffed olive 5

ONIONS
Per 28g/1oz unless otherwise stated

Raw	7
Boiled	4
Fried	98
Onion rings in batter, fried	145
Dried, per 15ml/1 level tablespoon	10
Fried, per 15ml/1 level tablespoon	25
Whole medium onion, raw, 75g/3oz	20
Pickled onion, each	5
Cocktail onion, each	1
Spring onion, each	3

ORANGES

Flesh only, per 28g/1oz	10
Flesh with skin, per 28g/1oz	7
Whole fruit, small, 150g/5oz	35
Whole fruit, medium, 225g/8oz	60
Whole fruit, large, 275g/10oz	75

ORANGE JUICE
Per 28ml/1floz

Sweetened	14
Unsweetened	11

OXTAIL

Stewed, without bone, per 28g/1oz	69
On the bone, stewed and skimmed of fat, per 28g/1oz	26

OYSTERS

With shells, raw, per 28g/1oz	2
Without shells, raw, per 28g/1oz	14
Per oyster	5

PARSLEY

Fresh, per 28g/1oz	6
Parsley sauce, per 15ml/1 level tablespoon	45

PARSNIPS
Per 28g/1oz

Raw	14
Boiled	16
Roast	30

PARTRIDGE

Roast, on bone, per 28g/1oz	36
Roast, meat only, per 28g/1oz	60

PASSION FRUIT

Flesh only, per 28g/1oz	10
With skin, per 28g/1oz	4

PASTA
Per 28g/1oz

White, raw, all shapes	105
White, boiled, all shapes	33
Wholewheat, raw, all shapes	95
Wholewheat, boiled, all shapes	34

PASTRY
Per 28g/1oz

Choux, raw	61
Choux, baked	95
Flaky, raw	120
Flaky, baked	160
Shortcrust, raw	130
Shortcrust, baked	150
Wholemeal, raw	125
Wholemeal, baked	145

PAW PAW OR PAPAYA

Canned, per 28g/1oz	18
Fresh, flesh only, per 28g/1oz	11

PEACHES

Canned in syrup, per 28g/1oz	25
Canned, half peach, drained	25
Canned in natural juice, per 28g/1oz	13
Fresh, with stones, per 28g/1oz	9
Whole fruit, 115g/4oz	35

PEANUTS
Per 28g/1oz unless otherwise stated

Shelled, fresh	162
Dry roasted	160
Roasted and salted	162
Peanut butter	177
Peanut butter, per 5ml/1 level teaspoon	35
Per peanut	5

PEARS
Per 28g/1oz unless otherwise stated

Cooking pears, raw, peeled	10
Dessert pears	8
Canned in syrup	22
Canned in syrup, drained, per half pear	30
Canned in natural juice, per 28g/1oz	11
Whole fruit, 150g/5oz	40

PEAS
Per 28g/1oz

Fresh, raw	19
Frozen, raw	15
Canned, garden	13
Canned, processed	23
Dried, raw	81
Dried, boiled	29
Split, raw	88
Split, boiled	34

Per 15ml/1 level tablespoon

Dried, boiled	30
Fresh or frozen, boiled	10
Pease pudding	35

PECAN

Per nut	15

PEPPER

Powdered, per pinch	0

PEPPERS (PIMENTOS)

Red or green, per 28g/1oz	4
Average pepper, 150g/5oz	20

PERCH

White, raw, per 28g/1oz	35
Yellow, raw, per 28g/1oz	25

PHEASANT

Meat only, roast, per 28g/1oz	60
On the bone, roast, per 28g/1oz	38

PIGEON

Meat only, roast, per 28g/1oz	65
On the bone, roast, per 28g/1oz	29

PIKE

Raw, per 28g/1oz	25

PILCHARDS

Canned in tomato sauce, per 28g/1oz	36

PIMENTOS

Canned in brine, drained, per 28g/1oz	6

PINEAPPLES

Canned in natural juice, per 28g/1oz	15
Canned in syrup, per 28g/1oz	22
Fresh, flesh only, per 28g/1oz	13
Slice of fresh pineapple, weighed with skin and core, 150g/5oz	35
Ring of canned, drained pineapple in syrup	35
Ring of canned, drained pineapple in natural juice	20
Ring of canned, drained pineapple in syrup, fried in batter	65

PINE KERNELS

Per 28g/1oz	180

PISTACHIO NUTS

Shelled, per 28g/1oz	180
Per nut	5

PLAICE
Per 28g/1oz unless otherwise stated

Fillet, raw or steamed	26
Fillet, in batter, fried	79
Fillet, in breadcrumbs, fried	65
Whole fillet in breadcrumbs, fried, 175g/6oz uncoated weight	435

PLANTAIN
Per 28g/1oz

Green, raw	32
Green, boiled	35
Ripe, fried	76

PLUMS
Per 28g/1oz unless otherwise stated

Cooking plums with stones, stewed without sugar	6
Cooking plums, with stones	7
Fresh dessert plums, with stones	10
Victoria dessert plum, each	15

POLLACK

On the bone, raw, per 28g/1oz	25

POLONY

Per 28g/1oz	80

POMEGRANATE

Flesh only, per 28g/1oz	20
Whole pomegranate, 200g/7oz	65

POPCORN

Per 28g/1oz	110

PORK
Per 28g/1oz unless otherwise stated

Belly rashers, raw, lean and fat	108
Belly rashers, grilled, lean and fat	113
Fillet (tenderloin), raw, lean only	42
Leg, raw, lean and fat, weighed without bone	76
Leg, raw, lean only, weighed without bone	42
Leg, roast, lean and fat	81
Leg, roast, lean only	52
Crackling	190
Scratchings	185
Fat from roast pork	150

Crackling, average portion, 10g/⅛oz	65
Pork chop, well grilled, 185g/6½oz raw weight	240
Pork chop, well fried, 185g/6½oz raw weight	290

POTATOES
Per 28g/1oz unless otherwise stated

Raw, peeled	25
Baked, weighed with skin	24
Boiled, old potatoes	23
Boiled, new potatoes	22
Canned, new potatoes, drained	15
Chips (average thickness)	70
Chips (crinkle cut)	80
Chips (thick cut)	40
Chips (thin cut)	85
Crisps	150
Roast, large chunks	40
Roast, medium chunks	45
Roast, small chunks	50
Sauté	40
Instant mashed potato powder, per 15ml/1 level tablespoon, dry	40
Jacket-baked potato, 200g/7oz raw weight	170
Jacket-baked potato with 15g/½oz knob butter	275
Mashed potato, 150g/5oz raw weight, mashed with 45ml/3 tablespoons skimmed milk	140
Mashed potato, 150g/5oz raw weight, mashed with 45ml/3 tablespoons Silver Top milk and 7g/¼oz knob butter	205
Roast potato, medium chunk, 45g/1¾oz	75

PRAWNS

With shells, per 28g/1oz	12
Without shells, per 28g/1oz	30
Per shelled prawn	2

PRUNES
Per 28g/1oz unless otherwise stated

Dried, no stones	46
Stewed, with stones, no sugar	21
Prune juice	25
Per prune	10

PUMPKIN

Flesh only, raw, per 28g/1oz	4
Pumpkin seeds, seed coat removed, per 28g/1oz	173

QUAIL

Raw, flesh only	37
Whole quail, raw, with skin, 115g/4oz	105
Whole quail, raw, without skin, 115g/4oz whole weight	65

QUINCES

Flesh only, raw, per 28g/1oz	7

RABBIT
Per 28g/1oz

Meat only, raw	35
Meat only, stewed	51
On the bone, stewed	26

RADISHES

Fresh, per 28g/1oz	4
Per radish	2

RAISINS

Dried, per 28g/1oz	70
Per 15ml/1 level tablespoon	25

RASPBERRIES

Fresh or frozen, per 28g/1oz	7
Canned, drained, per 28g/1oz	25

REDCURRANTS

Fresh, per 28g/1oz	6
Redcurrant jelly, per 5ml/1 level teaspoon	15

RHUBARB

Raw, per 28g/1oz	2
Stewed without sugar, per 28g/1oz	2

RICE

Brown, raw, per 28g/1oz	99
White, raw, per 28g/1oz	102
Boiled, per 28g/1oz	35

Per 15ml/1 level tablespoon

Boiled	20
Fried	35
Raw	35

ROCK

Seaside rock, per 28g/1oz	95

ROSE HIP SYRUP

per 28g/1oz	65
Per 15ml/1 tablespoon	45

ROYAL ICING

Per 28g/1oz	85

SAGO

Raw, per 28g/1oz	101

SAITHE (Coley)
Per 28g/1oz

Fillet, raw	21
Fillet, steamed	28
On the bone, steamed	24

SALMON
Per 28g/1oz

Canned	44
Fillet, steamed	56
On the bone, steamed	45
Smoked	40

SALSIFY

Boiled, per 28g/1oz	5

SALT

Per 28g/1oz	0

SARDINES

Canned in oil, drained, per 28g/1oz	62
Canned in tomato sauce, per 28g/1oz	50

SAUERKRAUT

Canned, per 28g/1oz	5

SAUSAGES
Each

Beef chipolata, well grilled	50
Beef large, well grilled	120
Beef skinless, well grilled	65
Pork chipolata, well grilled	65
Pork large, well grilled	125
Pork skinless, well grilled	95
Pork & beef chipolata, well grilled	125
Pork & beef large, well grilled	125

SAUSAGEMEAT

Per 28g/1oz, raw	80

SCALLOPS

Steamed, without shells, per 28g/1oz	30

SCAMPI

Fried in breadcrumbs, per 28g/1oz	90
Peeled, raw, per 28g/1oz	30

SEAKALE

Boiled, per 28g/1oz	2

SEMOLINA

Raw, per 28g/1oz	99
Per 15ml/1 level tablespoon	35

SESAME SEEDS

Per 28g/1oz	168

SHRIMPS
Per 28g/1oz

Canned, drained	27
Fresh, with shells	11
Fresh, without shells	33

SKATE

Fillet in batter, fried, per 28g/1oz	57

SMELTS

Without bones, fried, per 28g/1oz	115

SNAILS

Flesh only, per 28g/1oz	25

SOLE (DOVER)
Per 28g/1oz

Fillet, raw	23
Fillet, fried	61
Fillet, steamed or poached	26
On the bone, steamed or poached	18

SOLID VEGETABLE OIL

Per 28g/1oz	255

SOY SAUCE

Per 28g/1oz	20
Per 15ml/1 tablespoon	13

SPAGHETTI

Raw, per 28g/1oz	107
Wholewheat, raw, per 28g/1oz	97
Boiled, per 28g/1oz	33
Canned in tomato sauce, per 28g/1oz	17

SPINACH

Boiled, per 28g/1oz	9
Raw, per 28g/1oz	7

SPRATS

Fried without heads, per 28g/1oz	110

SPRING GREENS

Boiled, per 28g/1oz	3

SPRING ONIONS

Raw, per 28g/1oz	10
1 spring onion	3

SQUID

Flesh only, raw, per 28g/1oz	25

STRAWBERRIES

Fresh or frozen, per 28g/1oz	7
Canned, drained, per 28g/1oz	23

STURGEON

On the bone, raw, per 28g/1oz	25

SUET

Block, per 28g/1oz	255
Shredded, per 28g/1oz	235
Shredded, per 15ml/1 level tablespoon	85

SUGAR
White, brown, Demarara, icing, caster or granulated, per 28g/1oz	112
Per 5ml/1 level teaspoon	17
Large sugar lump	20
Small sugar lump	10

SULTANAS
Dried, per 28g/1oz	71
Per 15ml/1 level tablespoon	25

SUNFLOWER SEEDS
Per 28g/1oz, coat removed	170

SUNFLOWER SEED OIL
Per 28g/1oz	255

SWEDES
Raw, per 28g/1oz	6
Boiled, per 28g/1oz	5

SWEETBREADS
Lamb, raw, per 28g/1oz	37
Lamb, fried, per 28g/1oz	65

SWEETCORN
Canned in brine, per 28g/1oz	22
Canned, per 15ml/1 level tablespoon	10
Fresh, kernels only, boiled, per 28g/1oz	35
Frozen, per 28g/1oz	25
Whole medium cob	155

SWEET POTATO
Raw, per 28g/1oz	26
Boiled, per 28g/1oz	24

SWEETS
Per 28g/1oz unless otherwise stated
Barley sugar	100
Boiled sweets	93
Butterscotch	115
Filled chocolates	130
Fudge	111
Liquorice Allsorts	89
Marshmallows	90
Nougat	110
Peppermints	110
Toffee	122
Cough sweet, boiled, each	10
Cough pastille, each	5

SYRUPS
Per 28g/1oz
Golden	84
Maple	70

Per 15ml/1 level tablespoon
Golden	60
Maple	50

TANGERINES
Flesh only, per 28g/1oz	10
Flesh with skin, per 28g/1oz	7
Whole fruit, 75g/3oz	20

TAPIOCA
Dry, per 28g/1oz	102

TARAMASALATA
Per 28g/1oz	135

TEA
All brands, per cup, no milk or sugar	0

TOMATOES
Per 28g/1oz unless otherwise stated
Raw	4
Canned	3
Fried, halved	20
Fried, sliced	30
Chutney	44
Ketchup	28
Purée	19
Whole medium tomato, 50g/2oz	8

Per 15ml/1 level tablespoon
Ketchup	15
Purée	10
Tomato juice, 115ml/4floz	25

TONGUE
Per 28g/1oz
Lamb's, raw	55
Lamb's, stewed	82
Ox, boiled	83

TREACLE
Black, per 28g/1oz	73
Per 15ml/1 level tablespoon	50

TRIPE
Dressed, per 28g/1oz	17
Stewed, per 28g/1oz	28

TROUT
Fillet, smoked, per 28g/1oz	38
On the bone, poached or steamed, per 28g/1oz	25
Whole smoked trout, 160g/5½oz	150
Whole trout, poached or grilled without fat, 175g/6oz raw weight	150

TUNA
Per 28g/1oz
Canned in brine, drained	30
Canned in oil	82
Canned in oil, drained	60

TURKEY
Per 28g/1oz
Meat only, raw	30
Meat only, roast	40
Meat and skin, roast	48
Turkey ham joint, roast	35
Turkey ham joint, sliced and grilled	40
Roast, with skin and stuffing	50

TURNIPS
Raw, per 28g/1oz	6
Boiled, per 28g/1oz	4

VANILLA ESSENCE
Per 28g/1oz	0

VEAL
Per 28g/1oz unless otherwise stated
Cutlet, fried in egg and breadcrumbs	61
Fillet, raw	31
Fillet, roast	65
Escalope, fried in egg and breadcrumbs, 75g/3oz raw, uncoated weight	310

VENISON
Roast, meat only, per 28g/1oz	56

VINEGAR
Per 28ml/1floz	1

WALNUTS
Shelled, per 28g/1oz	149
Per walnut half	15

WATERCHESTNUTS
Per 28g/1oz	25

WATERCRESS
Per 28g/1oz	4

WATERMELON
Flesh only, per 28g/1oz	6
Flesh with skin, per 28g/1oz	3

WHEATGERM
Per 28g/1oz	100
Per 15ml/1 level tablespoon	18

WHELKS
With shells, boiled, per 28g/1oz	4
Without shells, boiled, per 28g/1oz	26

WHITEBAIT
Fried, per 28g/1oz	149

WHITE PUDDING
As sold, per 28g/1oz	128

WHITING
Per 28g/1oz
Fillet, fried	54
Fillet, steamed	26
On the bone, fried	49
On the bone, steamed	18

WINKLES
With shells, boiled, per 28g/1oz	4
Without shells, boiled, per 28g/1oz	21

WORCESTERSHIRE SAUCE
Per 28ml/1floz	20
Per 15ml/1 tablespoon	13

YAMS
Raw, per 28g/1oz	37
Boiled, per 28g/1oz	34

YEAST
Fresh, per 28g/1oz	15
Dried, per 28g/1oz	48
Dried, per 5ml/1 level teaspoon	8

YOGURT
Low fat natural, per 28g/1oz	15
Low fat natural, per 15ml/1 level tablespoon	10

YORKSHIRE PUDDING
Cooked, per 28g/1oz	60

Basic Alcoholic Drinks

BEERS
Average value for all beers, per 283ml/½ pint unless otherwise stated

Bitter or Pale Ale	90
Brown Ale	85
Light or Mild Ale	75
Lager	85

CIDER
Average value per 283ml/½ pint

Dry	105
Sweet	120
Vintage	180

HOMEBREWED BEER
Average value for all home brewed beers, per 575ml/1 pint

Bitter, Brown or Light Ale	240

LIQUEURS
Per pub measure 25ml/⅙ gill

Advocaat	65
Baileys Original Irish Cream	85
Benedictine	90
Calvados	60
Chartreuse (green)	100
Cherry Brandy	60
Cointreau	85
Crème de Menthe	80
Drambuie	85
Galliano, Kummel, Strega and Tia Maria	75
Grand Marnier	80
Kirsch	50
Sisca Crème de Cassis	65

PORT
Per pub measure, 50ml/⅓ gill

Average value for all Ports	75

SHERRY
Per small schooner, 50ml/⅓ gill
Average values for all sherries

Dry Sherry	55
Medium Sherry	60
Cream Sherry	65

SPIRITS
Per pub measure, 25ml/⅛ gill

Brandy, Whisky (Scotch, Irish or Bourbon), Gin, Rum and Vodka	55
Tequila	50

VERMOUTH
Per pub measure, 50ml/⅓ gill

Dry	55
Sweet	80

WINES
Per average glass, 150ml/5floz
Average value for all wines

Dry White	95
Sparkling White	110
Sweet White	125
Rosé	100
Dry Red	100
Sweet Red	120
De-alcoholised wines	35

Index

General Index

Index of Recipes and Serving Suggestions